FACING FEAR
A Young Woman's Personal Account of Surviving Breast Cancer

FACING FEAR
A Young Woman's Personal Account of Surviving Breast Cancer

Nancy Mikaelian Madey

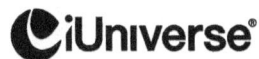

FACING FEAR

A Young Woman's Personal Account of Surviving Breast Cancer

iUniverse books may be ordered through booksellers or by contacting:

iUniverse
1663 Liberty Drive
Bloomington, IN 47403
www.iuniverse.com
1-800-Authors (1-800-288-4677)

Because of the dynamic nature of the Internet, any web addresses or links contained in this book may have changed since publication and may no longer be valid. The views expressed in this work are solely those of the author and do not necessarily reflect the views of the publisher, and the publisher hereby disclaims any responsibility for them.

ISBN: 978-0-5951-5117-2 (sc)
ISBN: 978-1-4697-5093-4 (e)

Print information available on the last page.

iUniverse rev. date: 09/10/2019

To my husband Randy,

my son David Tod,

and my newly born daughter, Nicole Alice, who will be aware of, and hopefully never experience the fear of breast cancer.

Also included in this dedication are those women who have fought the battle of breast cancer with strength and courage.

Acknowledgements

Special thanks to the following people for their love,
support, and prayers:

Kathryn Mitchell and Sally Newall who spent countless hours editing and proofing my manuscript.

Those who contributed to the "Perspectives" section of this book: my husband, my mother, my brother and sister, Mary Laros, and Kathryn Mitchell. Thank you for sharing your personal thoughts and feelings for this publication.

My husband Randy for holding my hand each step of the way and loving me unconditionally. Thank you for your patience, understanding, and continued support which enabled me to write my story.

David and Nicole, my precious son and daughter, who make my life more meaningful. Thank you for bestowing joy on our family.

My loving mother who traveled from Wisconsin to California several times to be with me throughout my cancer ordeal. It was comforting to have you by my side. You made me realize that I'm never too old to be nurtured.

My late father who modeled his extraordinary fight with cancer and set an example for me to follow.

My brother Tod C. Mikaelian and sister Kathy Merrick who I know I can always count on.

Dr. Sam Mikaelian, an uncle who is like a father to me. Thank you for counseling me through difficult times and helping me put my emotions into proper perspective. And, for the additional medical opinions you sought—for this, I am truly grateful.

My family and relatives: Anne Lemberger, Tom and Virginia Herbst, Bob and Mary Zauner, Kay and Catherine Mikaelian, Andrew and Marcy Mikaelian, George and Mimi Schwabe, Harry and Shari Esayian, John and Sue Esayian, Don and Leslie Nelson, Craig and Jean Azizian, Tony and Karen Ferraro, Dr. Richard and Betty Madey, Louise Madey, Drs. Sheldon and Doren Pinnell, Richard and Diane Foote, Saul and Daryl Gomez, Rick and Terri Madey, Ron and Kathy Madey, Paul Kirch, and all of my aunts, uncles, cousins, nieces, nephews, friends, neighbors, and those around the world who I have never met who prayed for my strength and recovery.

Kathryn Mitchell who is more than a friend—thank you for teaching me that I have the power within myself to overcome just about anything.

Judy Jonsson, for sharing her breast cancer experience with me. Thank you for walking me through my double mastectomy and the various stages of breast reconstruction. You helped turn a negative experience into a positive one.

The spiritual support from Father Yeprem Keligian and the congregation of St. Mesrob Armenian Apostolic Church in Racine, Wis., Pastor Tim McCalmont and the congregation at the Presbyterian Church of the Covenant in Costa Mesa, Calif., and special prayers and spiritual enlightenment from Toni Brosius, Jon Roberts, and Rose Kaprelian.

My best friends Mary Laros, Edna Parish and Sandi Glisper who always fill my heart with joy and laughter.

The late Irene Josephson, Candy Connors-Yankowy, Dean and Julie Page, Kevin and Kristy Reiser, Dr. Deborah Pauer-Salaben and Matthew Salaben, and Clara Escobar for their friendship and kindness, and Lisa Ennis for her listening ear.

My co-workers: Kathryn Mitchell, Laura Prater, Marica Willett, Maria Rosa-Madruga, Victoria Chaisson, Judy Quenzer, Susan Duggin, and Paula Brichaux who lived my experience with me. Janet Clancy, Rick Sbrocca, and David Dukes for taking a special interest in my well-being.

I am deeply grateful to the team of highly intelligent doctors who cared for me: Dr. Kenneth Kraus, for saving my life through early breast cancer detection; Dr. C.H. Baick, for his magnificent surgical skills, and sound medical recommendations; Dr. Tariq Mahmood and Dr. Neil Barth, for their highly respected medical opinions; Dr. Ernest Ngo for his knowledge and expertise in the areas of Diagnostic Imaging and Radiation Oncology; Dr. Pamela Botzbach for her expertise in anesthesiology; Dr. Mark Krugman, for guiding me through the breast reconstruction process and achieving a fabulous end result; and Dr. Samuel Carlis, my family physician, for his expert medical advice and recommendations.

Special thanks to Dr. Kraus' medical staff, namely Terry Braun; the medical staff at the Comprehensive Breast Health Center in Santa Ana, Calif., namely Margo Materie, Earlene Hogan, and Alice Rodriquez; the medical staff at Dr. Krugman's office, namely Laurie Schwabe and Christine Chen; the staff technicians at West Coast Radiology Center in Santa Ana, Calif., namely Bill Braggins, Ramin Daryabary, and Annemarie Lynch; and the medical staff at Western Medical Center in Santa Ana, Calif.

And, thank you God, for allowing me the gift of life and helping to enrich my spirituality in a way I never imagined. Moreover, thank you for blessing us with our son David and the newest addition to our family, Nicole Alice born on April 11, 2000—just one year after completing my breast reconstruction.

Prologue

Some things are hard to understand. Five months after giving birth to our beautiful son David Tod, I was diagnosed with breast cancer. I was only 35.

My husband Randy and I had been married for two and a half years, and just became parents for the first time. Our life with little David was merely beginning. I certainly didn't want my life to come to an end—not then anyway.

I've heard it said, "Life is what happens when you're busy making other plans." How true that is. I had a lot of plans: Plans to rock our baby in my arms, plans to walk to school with him on his first day of kindergarten, plans to teach him how to ride a bicycle, and later teach him how to drive a car, plans to see him graduate from high school and college, plans to see him get married, and one day rock *his* baby in my arms. Those were the plans.

Contracting breast cancer was one of the furthest things from my mind, and one of the last things I could have ever imagined. I didn't know how or why this could have happened, as I understood that "mammograms are not necessary for women under 40 years of age, unless there is a family history." Fitting into neither of those categories, I never dreamed it could happen to me.

My doctor informed me that one out of every 622 women 35 years old get this disease. It just so happened I was the *one*. It's funny because

I know that if I were to play the lottery with odds like that I would have never won!

I learned that breast cancer can be hereditary, and women with a family history have a higher risk of getting the disease. That's what bothered me the most—I have no family history of breast cancer and I come from a family with generations that are predominately female. I later learned that having breast cancer in your family may increase your risk, however, approximately 70 percent to 80 percent of the women who are diagnosed with it do not have a family history of breast cancer. Go figure!

The word *cancer* was familiar to me, as I had just lost my father to lymphoma two years prior. I witnessed his battle with cancer for 14 months as he struggled to do everything humanly possible to stay alive—up to and including chemotherapy and experimental treatments. I saw how he went from a picture of wholesome health to a weak, helpless shell of a man.

Was I now headed down that same road? Who would take care of my son? How would my husband cope with this? How would I break the news to my mother, who was still grieving the loss of her husband of 48 years? How would my two siblings and my relatives react? Thousands of thoughts began entering my mind like a revolving door.

My life was changing before my eyes. Little did I know, this was only the beginning....

1

It was November 19, 1996 when I went to see my gynecologist, Dr. Kraus, for my first routine examination after David was born. He examined my breasts and found a lump on the right side.

"Do you feel that?" he asked guiding my fingertips to the lump.

"Yes, now that you point it out. It's so small. I would have never detected it on my own," I said.

"It could be a cyst or a clogged milk duct from breast feeding. How old are you?" he asked.

"I'm 35."

"Nancy, I'd like you to have a mammogram. It's probably nothing, but I want to be sure," he said.

Since Randy was away on a business trip, I told a few of my close friends at work about the lump. They assured me that it was probably nothing, and told me it was not uncommon for women to develop cysts in their breasts.

That night Randy called. I told him about the lump Dr. Kraus found. Randy didn't seem overly concerned—he needed to have more facts before he would allow his emotions to enter the equation. I have always admired that about him.

The next day I went for the mammogram. It was my first time having one, so I didn't quite know what to expect. I was extremely calm and very confident that this lump was nothing to be alarmed about. I knew several women who had lumps in their breasts that turned out to be nothing but cysts.

When my name was called the technician escorted me to a small dressing room, told me to undress from the waist up and handed me a hospital gown. From there I was led to another room for the mammogram. I had heard horror stories about how painful and uncomfortable mammograms can be, so I was prepared.

While standing, the technician lifted my right breast up to a cold metal plate. She pushed a few buttons to align the positioning as another plate came down flattening my breast like a pancake. She told me to take a deep breath and left the room as she took the x-ray. She repeated the procedure on my left breast.

A few minutes later she came back and said she needed to take another x-ray of the right side—the breast with the lump.

"Why?" I asked.

"The radiologist requested a magnification," she said.

At this point, I started to think that something could be wrong. I tried probing the technician and asked her a few questions.

"Is it a cyst?" She didn't answer and repositioned me for the next x-ray.

"Is it cancer?" I asked with even more concern. She continued to evade my questions.

"Sometimes we don't get a good picture and we need to re-do the x-ray. We'll know more in a few minutes," she said.

I sat down and waited patiently for her to tell me that everything was fine, and I could go home. I tried to reassure myself that the lump was just a cyst and there was nothing to worry about.

Two minutes seemed like two hours. The longer I waited for the results, the harder it was for me not to engage in the "what if" game. I began having a dialogue with myself inside my head.

"What if it's cancer?

Naaaah. I'm too young for that.

But, what if it is?

Well, then they'll just take the lump out!

Yeah, that's pretty simple."

Before I could continue the rest of my conversation, the technician came back and said that the radiologist wanted to perform an ultrasound to get a closer look at the lump.

My stomach turned inside out and my heart pounded. The technician introduced me to the radiologist and asked me to lie down on an examination table. He began rolling an electronic wand over the breast in question, while looking at a computerized screen.

"My gynecologist suspects it's a cyst or a clogged milk duct," I said as he continued staring at the screen. "What do you see?" I asked.

"Well, it's definitely not a cyst or a clogged milk duct. I suggest that you have a biopsy taken."

My heart stopped as fear engulfed me. I started trembling as tears streamed down my face and the panic took hold. Oh my God!

My voice crackled as I exclaimed, "This can't be cancer, I have a five-month-old baby!"

"We won't know what it is until the biopsy is performed," he said calmly.

As I left the office with tears in my eyes, I was handed some pamphlets about breast cancer. Why on earth would I be given these pamphlets if they didn't think I had breast cancer? I went outside and literally ran to my gynecologist's office just a few doors away. With tears rolling down my cheeks, I opened the office door to find an empty waiting room and Terry, Dr. Kraus' nurse, behind the receptionist desk.

"Thank God you're here Terry," I said leaning over the receptionist's counter. Terry had been Dr. Kraus's nurse for over ten years and I had gotten to know her quite well. In a state of sheer frenzy, I told her what had just happened, and showed her the literature I was given. She was very compassionate and told me that Dr. Kraus was not in the office but she would contact him to let him know. In the meantime, she made an appointment for me to see Dr. Baick, a surgical oncologist at the Comprehensive Breast Health Center, for the following day. Terry told me that Dr. Baick was an excellent surgeon and not to worry. She handed me an order for a needle biopsy.

I was numb. I walked out to the parking lot in a daze. I got in my car and drove to my office. My head was in another world. I debated whether or not I should even go to work, but felt an urgency to share the news with a few of my female colleagues. I knew they would give me the support I so badly needed.

When I arrived at the office, the majority of the department was away on business attending the same trade show as my husband. I had just put my briefcase down on my desk when Maria and Laura, two of my colleagues, called from the trade show to find out how my doctor's appointment went.

I spoke with Maria first—she seemed very surprised to learn just how serious my situation had become. She tried comforting me but seemed at a loss for words—she handed the phone to Laura.

I could tell Laura was concerned, too. She said she was flying home that night, and offered to accompany me to my doctor's appointment. I found a great deal of comfort in knowing that I wouldn't have to go alone. We ironed out the details and she said she'd pick me up from the office at 9 a.m. the following morning.

The remainder of my workday was emotionally draining. As much as I tried to concentrate on my work, I couldn't. I became preoccupied with the thought that I could possibly have breast cancer.

When Randy called that evening, I told him everything that had happened and why I needed to have a biopsy taken.

"Do you want me to fly home tonight so I can be with you?" he asked.

"No, that's okay. Laura is going to go to the doctor's office with me. If it turns out to be something major, I'll call you."

The next morning I drove to work in the fog and rain, which only added to my gloomy state. Laura picked me up from work at 9 a.m., as planned, and we headed for the breast center.

Laura understood how I was feeling. She had discovered a lump in her breast a year earlier and had it removed. Thankfully, it ended up being a benign cyst. Although Laura is eight years my junior, I took solace in talking to her. She's a wonderful listener, a positive person, and someone I could always count on to help me keep things in perspective.

When we arrived at the breast center, we sat down. I was handed some paperwork to complete and before we knew it, I was called in. The nurse escorted me into an examination room and handed me a gown. She proceeded to take my blood pressure and then asked me a few questions. I slipped into the gown and within minutes Dr. Baick entered the room.

"What are you doing here? You're too young to be here!" I nervously chuckled and said, "Yes, I know."

He extended his hand and introduced himself. He asked me a few general questions and then requested I lie down so he could examine my breasts. He poked and prodded—not uttering a word. I was too scared to even ask what he thought. Then he told me I could sit up.

He pulled the films of my mammogram out of a large manila envelope and hung them over a light box. He stared and stared. Then he picked up a huge magnifying glass and looked even closer. The longer he looked, the more scared I became.

He turned around and said, "Nancy, I'm pretty sure this is cancer. Rather than doing a needle biopsy, I'm recommending that we perform a lumpectomy."

"How confident are you that the lump is cancerous?" I asked.

"I'm 80 percent sure," he said looking me straight in the eye. My heart dropped into my stomach. I'm sure he saw the fear in my face. I tried to hold back the tears, but couldn't.

"I have a five-month-old baby!" I exclaimed with my hands cupped to my face.

He reached out and touched my shoulder, "The lump is small and you're very fortunate that it's been detected early. You're not going to die!"

I found some comfort in his words, yet I couldn't help but feel that a portion of my future was being stolen from me.

His nurse asked if I would like my friend to come in. I nodded yes. When Laura entered the room, I introduced her to Dr. Baick and she sat down in one of the guest chairs. The nurse asked me for my insurance card and said she would set me up for surgery.

"Can you schedule the operation as soon as possible? I don't want this lump in my body any longer than it has to be!"

"I'll see what I can do," she said.

I turned to Laura and said, "Dr. Baick thinks it's cancer."

"You've got to be kidding me!" she exclaimed.

"We'll know more once the lump is removed," said Dr. Baick. "We need to first find out if it's cancer, and if so, whether it's invasive or non-invasive. There are two types of cancer," he explained, "those that invade the body by multiplying and traveling through the lymph nodes (invasive), and those that do not (non-invasive)."

At this point I felt so overwhelmed that I couldn't absorb the information. I wasn't even sure how much of what the doctor just told me I had retained!

Just then the nurse came back and said that she was able to schedule me for outpatient surgery the following morning, November 22nd, at 7:30 a.m. However, I had to be at the hospital an hour and a half prior—that meant 6 a.m. She gave me a list of directions to follow, an order to have blood drawn at the adjacent hospital, and her card with the number of a 24-hour answering service to call if I had any questions. I thanked her for her kindness, got dressed and walked to the hospital with Laura.

I was so thankful that Laura was with me. She was one of the many key people whose strength I grew to depend on. I was anxious to go back home and call Randy. I knew he'd come home right away once he knew I was going to have an operation. It was a five-and-one-half-hour drive, and with the rain it could take longer.

2

It was pouring down rain when Laura and I left the breast center. We stared out the clear glass door waiting for the rain to let up. Laura put her arm around my shoulder as we stood listening to the raindrops hitting the pavement.

"You're going to be fine," she said.

"I think I need time to process everything that just happened," I said.

"I feel numb. I'm obviously not in any condition to go back to work. I won't be able to concentrate."

"I can take the rest of the day off and stay with you until Randy gets home," she offered.

"Would you? I really don't want to be alone right now," I said with tears in my eyes. "I'm counting on you to lift my spirits!"

We opened our umbrellas and dashed outside to the parking lot. Still feeling numb and in a state of disbelief, I got in Laura's Jeep and she drove me back to work to pick up my car. I led the way as Laura followed me home.

When we arrived, I immediately paged Randy to our telephone number. Within minutes the phone rang.

"Hello."

"I just got your page. Is everything okay?"

Just hearing Randy's voice made me cry. "No," I said sniffling. "I'm having surgery tomorrow morning to get the lump removed—the specialist suspects it's cancer."

"I don't believe it!"

"Neither do I. It feels so surreal. Do you think you'll be able to come home tonight?" I asked.

"I'm sure that won't be a problem. I'll try to be home before 10 p.m. and we can talk more then, okay? I love you."

"I love you too," I said and hung up the phone.

It was now going on 1 p.m. and neither Laura nor I had had lunch.

"Could you go for some pizza?" I asked.

I ordered a large pepperoni pizza and we played with David on the living room floor until it was delivered. I found comfort holding David in my arms—especially after the emotionally draining day I just had.

David is my life. I need him as much as he needs me. I refused to allow breast cancer to stand in the way of being his mother.

David was an adorable little baby with soft brown wavy hair and big brown eyes—features that Randy and I possess. In fact, it's not difficult to tell that David is our son—he's a nice mixture of both of us. When the baby sitter put David down for his afternoon nap, I called my brother Tod who lives down the street from us, and my sister Kathy, who lives in Colorado, to tell them that I was scheduled to have a lumpectomy the following day. I made arrangements with Tod to take care of David the morning of my operation until the baby sitter arrived.

I asked my siblings not to tell our mother about the lump or the lumpectomy. I wanted to tell her myself—in person. She was scheduled to fly out in a few days to spend the Thanksgiving holiday with us. I planned to explain everything to her when she arrived. I didn't want her to worry more than she needed to. Strange as it may seem, I was more concerned about how my loved ones would react to hearing the potential cancer diagnosis than I was about myself. I didn't want *anyone* to worry.

I tried to stay composed while we were eating, but Laura could tell that I was starting to feel scared and uneasy. "Nancy," she blurted out, "we don't even know if you have cancer yet. It's just Dr. Baick's educated guess."

Laura had a point. This was not the time to fall apart. I had to stay calm until I had all of the facts. In less than 24 hours I would know more. We watched TV and talked openly about the cancer diagnosis. Whenever I'd mention a negative thought, she'd strip away the fear by replacing it with a positive one. Laura, did indeed, lift my spirits!

By 9:30 p.m. Randy was home. I greeted him with a hug and a kiss and felt an instant sense of security, knowing that I didn't have to face this alone. Once Randy got settled, he sat down and joined us in the living room. Laura and I filled him in on the conversations we had had with Dr. Baick and his staff. Randy was very level-headed and agreed with Laura, that we really shouldn't jump to any conclusions until we had all of the facts. In my mind, however, I had to begin preparing for the worst, but was ready to be pleasantly surprised if the lump turned out to be benign.

As Laura was getting ready to go home, she offered to meet Randy at the hospital the following morning and wait with him until I was out of surgery. We agreed that it was a good idea, and thanked her for being such a wonderful friend.

That night my mind began flooding with negative thoughts, making it difficult for me to fall asleep. Randy snuggled up next to me and held me tightly. He kept reassuring me that I was going to be fine; but I found it difficult to believe.

Tears rolled down my face onto my pillow as I began thinking about my father. I remembered how strong and brave he was when he was first diagnosed with cancer. He fought this disease with determination and dignity. I wanted to do the same.

The alarm went off at 5:15 a.m. I felt tired and anxious. Maybe a shower will help me wake up and calm my nerves, I thought. With my eyes half-closed, I opened the shower door, stepped in, and slowly turned on the faucet. Thoughts of my father's cancer experience continued to fill my head. I needed to talk to him—even if it was just a one-sided conversation. I wanted him to know what I was going through.

"Dad," I said. "I'm so scared. I'm having surgery in a few hours. My doctor thinks I have breast cancer. Please watch over me and help me get through this. Even though you're not here, you're still my dad and I need you." At least one of my parents *know*, I thought. The other will find out tomorrow.

My morning routine was fast and simple as I was instructed not to eat breakfast, and not to wear any make-up. I was also told to wear loose, comfortable clothing. As I stepped out of the shower, I recalled my mother giving me one of my dad's favorite sweat suits to remember him. I tucked it away in a dresser drawer two years ago. I'm going to wear his sweat suit, I thought. It's big, and I was told to wear something loose and comfortable—it will be perfect! I opened the dresser drawer and pulled it out. The jacket was teal and purple, with matching teal sweat pants. I hugged the jacket that I so vividly remember him wearing. My eyes welled with tears as I slipped my arms through the sleeves, and put on the sweat pants. I felt a part of my dad was with me, and I wasn't going into surgery alone. I opened my jewelry box and put a guardian angel pin on the collar—I felt doubly protected.

Randy was waiting for me downstairs in the living room with my brother Tod. When I came down the stairs they both recognized the sweat suit I was wearing. Neither of them said a word. I'm sure it was a rather eerie thing for them to see, but it was something I needed to do.

We arrived at the hospital five minutes early. We sat in the waiting room; Randy interlocked his fingers with mine. He held my hand tightly as he lowered his head to kiss the back of my hand.

"Everything's going to be okay," he whispered.

When my name was called, I followed the nurse into the patient prepping area. She handed me a gown to put on and told me which gurney to lie on. Although I was a little nervous about being anesthetized, I desperately wanted this operation to be over.

The anesthesiologist introduced himself and told me the types of drugs he would be using. The nurses began setting up the I.V., and asked if I would like to see my husband before I went into the operating room.

Within a minute, Randy was at my side, holding my hand and wiping away my tears. I am blessed to be married to such an affectionate and compassionate man. This is when I needed Randy the most, and I was so thankful that I wasn't going through this terrible ordeal alone.

"I'll see you when you wake up," he said as I was wheeled down the corridor.

The next thing I remember was waking up in the recovery room recalling that I was in the hospital getting a lump removed from my breast. I could hear the nurses talking among themselves as I dozed in and out of sleep. I also heard Dr. Baick's voice in the distance. I was somewhat groggy when he approached me on the gurney.

"Is it cancer?" I asked in a soft whisper. "Yes," he said nodding.

"Is it invasive?" I asked in another soft whisper.

"We won't know for approximately four more days. The pathologists have to run tests on the tissue—we'll have the results on Tuesday when you come in to see me," he said while gently patting my shoulder.

"What are the odds of it being invasive or non-invasive cancer?" I asked.

"It's 50-50. Just try to relax and rest," he said. "You can see your husband shortly."

Once I truly regained consciousness, I was wheeled to another area in the recovery room where Randy and Laura were waiting. Randy held my dad's sweat suit jacket in his hands and put it by the side of the bed. He had a beautiful arrangement of flowers with a cute little stuffed bear on the night stand. He stood over me looking into my eyes, stroking my forehead.

"How do you feel?" he asked.

"I feel pretty good, all things considered. I don't feel any pain—at least not yet," I replied.

Laura stood in the background and told me that I looked good for just having had surgery. I gazed down and saw a fairly large gauze bandage over the upper half of my right breast.

"It's cancerous you know," I blurted out looking at both of their faces.

"I know," said Randy, "Dr. Baick told me."

"What exactly did he say?" I curiously asked.

"He said we'd know more once we have the results of the pathology report. Then we'll review our options."

"Options?!" I exclaimed. "What options?"

Randy lowered his head and said, "Maybe a mastectomy."

"A mastectomy!" I screamed, as I grabbed my dad's sweat suit jacket and threw it at him.

Laura jumped in, "Nancy, you don't know anything yet—you're jumping to conclusions. Everything could be fine. We'll just have to wait and see."

"I want to see Dr. Baick!" I demanded, shouting loud enough for the nursing staff to hear me.

One of the nurses came running over. "What's the matter?" she asked.

"I just found out I have cancer and now I'm hearing that I may need a mastectomy!" I exclaimed as tears rolled down my face. "I want to see Dr. Baick," I demanded once again.

"Dr. Baick has left the hospital," the nurse said, "but I'll be more than happy to call his head nurse, Alice, to come and speak with you. She's Dr. Baick's right hand person who works closely with all of his cancer patients. Don't worry, today breast reconstructions are so realistic—one can't tell the difference."

"I'm not having my breast removed!" I screamed.

Randy and Laura sat speechless. How could I have been so naive? Why hadn't the possibility of a mastectomy ever crossed my mind? Having had no firsthand experience with this, I believed that if the lump was removed, the cancer was gone—end of story. It made perfect sense to me.

Just as I was concluding these thoughts, Alice came to my bedside. She calmly explained that the pathologist had to determine whether the cancer was invasive or non-invasive before any type of treatment could be recommended. I told Alice that my biggest fear was having to undergo chemotherapy treatments. The mere thought of having chemicals injected into my body that were powerful enough to make my hair fall out terrified me. I saw what my dad had gone through and I didn't want that happen to me. She told me that there were new oral forms of chemotherapy without the severe side affects, and I may not have to undergo that kind of therapy at all. I'm sure she could tell I was anticipating the worst.

Alice looked me squarely in the eye and said, "You're not going to die from this!"

"Tell me that one more time," I pleaded.

"You're NOT going to die."

I thanked her as she reached down to hug me. I felt somewhat better. Before she left, she gave me her business card and said that if I ever needed to talk to her, she had an answering service and would be available to me 24 hours a day, seven days a week. Having her card in my possession was the security I needed.

Randy encouraged me not to speculate. I found that easier said than done. I've always been the type of person who needed to be in control and have all of the answers. The thought of waiting FOUR DAYS to get test results that would determine my future was more than I was willing to handle. I didn't want my patience to be tried. I wanted to have the answers NOW!

I was scared. REALLY scared. I feared the unknown. I feared the future. I feared how my life was going to unfold, and how I would cope with the final outcome.

About an hour later, I was released to go home. Randy pulled our car around to the hospital exit as one of the nurses wheeled me out. I slept the duration of our 30-minute car ride home.

Randy helped me out of the car and walked me to the front door. Once inside the house, he assisted me up the stairs, step by step. I went in our son's room and peered down at him. He was sleeping ever so soundly—not a care in the world. He had no idea what his mother was going through. I was thankful for that. My main objective was to stay healthy so that I could provide for him.

Randy walked me to our bedroom, propped up some pillows for me to rest on and brought me some lunch. I hardly ate. All I could think about was how in a few short days, my life had changed. *How* it changed, and to *what degree* it changed was yet to be determined.

Later that afternoon, Laura and Marcia, my director from the office, stopped by to visit me. Marcia and I had worked together for several years and we'd grown very close. In fact, she was with me on a business trip when I learned that my dad passed away. She was very compassionate and supportive every step of the way. Marcia knew that I had been through a lot and was genuinely concerned about my well-being.

I was propped up in bed and Marcia sat beside me. I began telling her how frightened I was, and how scared I was to break the news to my mom. Since Marcia was a mother of two children close to my age, I asked her how she would take the news if she learned that one of them had cancer.

"Well, naturally, I would be upset," she said, "but you have to tell your mom—and when you do, you'll feel better. Your mother would want you to tell her." Marcia was right. She gave me a big hug and told me to call her any time I needed to talk.

After she left, I called my uncle Sam—my dad's younger brother who lives in Glenview, Illinois. Uncle Sam and I have been close since I was a little girl. However, after my dad passed away we became even closer—he's now like a father to me.

Uncle Sam has a Ph.D. in Guidance and Counseling and has always made himself available to me—both on a personal and professional level. For as long as I can remember, I would seek his professional advice and know that our conversations were kept in strict confidence. Hence, I knew it was time to call Uncle Sam and tell him about my situation. Moreover, I needed to seek out his professional opinion as to how I should tell my mother.

I explained what had transpired over the past few days and he listened attentively. He spoke in a very calm manner, which was extremely soothing to me. Perhaps that was his way of helping me rid my fears. He told me he knew of many women who had this disease and are now long-time survivors.

"You're going to be fine," he said. "I'm not worried and I don't want you to worry either."

In the back of my mind I knew he had to be worried—he just didn't want me to know it. He was trying to comfort and protect me like a father would.

Losing my dad was the most difficult thing I had ever experienced in my life—far worse than getting breast cancer. My dad was diagnosed with lymphoma in 1993, just months before Randy and I became engaged. My dad's serious health condition came as a shock since cancer didn't run in our family. Moreover, my dad's parents were still living—his father was 96 and his mother was 90.

I was devastated when I first heard the news. I can remember the evening my mom called to give me the news. My heart dropped as I held my stomach, wailing in pain. "This can't be true!" I cried. "Not dad!" I laid awake in bed the entire night, sobbing as I feared what my life would be like without him. I couldn't bear the thought—not even for a minute—yet it managed to consume my mind non-stop, causing me months of agony.

Fortunately, I was able to visit my parents quite often while in route on business. I felt spending time with my dad was the medicine he needed. I would notice changes in him each time I saw him. Some visits he looked better than others. However, in spite of all of the physical changes attributed to chemotherapy treatments, my dad still kept his humor. I can remember sitting outside chatting with him in the backyard when he pulled a handful of this thick curly hair from his head and said, "Look Nancy, it's starting to fall out now." He released his hair into the gust of wind and said, "Some lucky bird will be able to build a nice home with it!"

Randy and I decided to have our wedding in Wisconsin to make it easier for everyone. My parents offered to make all of our arrangements including securing the church, the hotel, the band, etc. It was a good opportunity for them to focus on something other than my dad's health. I offered to move up our wedding date, but my dad wouldn't hear of it. "Nancy, I'm not going anywhere until I walk you down the aisle." Walking me down that aisle on our wedding date, May 29, 1994, became his goal.

By February and March of that year, my dad had been in and out of the hospital. He could no longer dress himself nor get out of a chair alone. He needed constant assistance.

My stress level was climbing to an all-time high. I was coming to the realization that my life was changing in more ways than one. I would be losing the man I loved most in this world and gaining another. I was entering a new chapter in my life. From that point on, I knew I would never be the same woman.

In early April, my mom called and told me that my dad had taken a turn for the worse. I knew it was time for me and Randy to fly to Wisconsin so my dad could witness our marriage. Randy agreed that it was the proper thing to do.

When we arrived at the hospital, I was shocked to see how rapidly my dad had deteriorated. He was suffering terribly and refused to let go. I fought back the tears as I held his hand and gave him permission to die. But it didn't matter—he was determined that he wasn't going anywhere until he walked me down the aisle just as he had promised. And so he did. The small service was performed in the hospital chapel on April 9th. Uncle Sam assisted my dad from behind as he proceeded to give me away to my future husband—the new man who would now love and care for me as he did.

I offered to spend the following few weeks with my dad, but he encouraged me to go back to California. "Your place is with your husband now. There's nothing more you can do for me," he said.

Saying goodbye to my dad was one of the hardest things I have ever done—I was saying goodbye forever. I knelt down at his bedside and held his hand. I told him what a wonderful father he was and how much I loved him. As tears rolled down our cheeks, he whispered back in a weak voice, "I love you—God be with you."

Twelve days after my wedding he passed away. However, on my wedding day, he made me promise that our May 29th wedding would still go on as planned, with or without him. We honored his wishes.

In his heart of hearts, he knew he wasn't going to see the elaborate Armenian wedding that he and my mother had arranged for Randy and me. Therefore, he had asked my uncle to walk me down the aisle on his behalf—which my uncle did. It was a bittersweet occasion.

I grieved endlessly, for months, wondering if and when I would ever be rid of the awful void that lingered deep inside. I even sought professional counseling to help me cope with the pain. I finally came to terms with his death and accepted his loss 18 months later. Although the pain has subsided, I still miss my dad tremendously.

We had such a special father-daughter relationship. That's why losing him was so difficult for me. One thing I knew for sure was that if he were still alive he would have been heartbroken to know I had breast cancer. I was sure my mom would be too when I told her. I needed the motherly love and nurturing support that only she could provide. Although I had only been a mother for five months, I was able to understand how devastating it would be to learn that her own child was diagnosed with cancer.

Uncle Sam advised me on how to break the news to her. "You need to be very strong and unemotional when you tell her, and be sure to deliver the message in a calm manner without tears. Crying will only make your mom feel worse and cause her to worry about you even more," he said. We talked a short while more, and before we hung up he said, "Remember, no tears." I wondered whether or not I would be capable of telling her without shedding a tear.

That night I tried to keep my mind busy by watching TV. I couldn't concentrate on anything. I was still trying to digest the fact that I had breast cancer—everything was happening so fast. Tuesday the lump was found; Wednesday was the mammogram; Thursday was my appointment with Dr. Baick and Friday, November 22nd, the lump was removed.

In four more days I would know what my future would hold. I kept wondering how I would be able to get through it. "One day at a time," I kept reminding myself—I now understood the true meaning of that phrase: We must learn to live in the moment. Still, the waiting was agonizing. I didn't know what to do next or where to turn.

I didn't feel comfortable sharing my fears with Randy because I knew he was scared, too. I needed to be strong for him, and felt guilty for causing my husband so much pain and sorrow. I could tell he was extremely concerned. I also knew he wanted to be my pillar of strength.

Although I'd been told I wasn't going to die, I couldn't help but feel that my life span had been shortened. Maybe I would only live to be 45 years old instead of 85, as I had hoped.

I tried to imagine what thoughts might be flowing through Randy's mind. *Did he think he would be a young widower? Did he wonder who would take care of David? Was he concerned with how David would get along without his mother, and how he would get along without his wife?*

Then I started wondering too, and tried answering the questions I was raising in my own mind. *"Yes, he would be a young widower. Who would take care of David? My mother? My sister or brother? One of Randy's sisters or brothers? Gosh, I need to write a will! Would he remarry? I guess I would want him to. Randy's still young and such a family-man—he deserves to continue to live his life as he would have with me. I love him enough to want that to happen. Besides, David would need a mother to care for him. I hope this woman would love David and care for him as much as I do. Perhaps he'd hire a baby sitter to care for David while he worked and a housekeeper to do his laundry, cook, and clean. Why am I doing this? Why am I projecting all of these situations and outcomes?"* It's amazing what the mind can do if you let it. And, I emphasize those words "if you let it." I was mentally exhausted!

That night Randy climbed into bed with me and wrapped his arms around my waist holding me ever so tightly. I felt safe and secure in his arms as I laid my head on the pillow and fell asleep.

3

The next morning when I awoke, my first thought was that I had breast cancer. Although I felt like it was a nightmare, this was my reality. I had tossed and turned most of the night, fearing the type of treatment I may need to undergo, as well as the possibilities of a reoccurrence or a new occurrence in the other breast. I laid in bed wondering how this could have happened to me. I led a clean and healthy life—I didn't smoke, drink, or use drugs. I became more concerned with wanting to find out *how* I got this disease rather than wondering, "why me?"

At 7 a.m. Clara, our baby sitter, came over to take care of David. I was told not to do any lifting after my operation—including lifting David. It broke my heart that I couldn't tend to my baby as any other new mother would. When he'd wake up from his naps, Clara would lie him in my lap, and I would gaze into his big brown eyes.

David was all the medicine I needed. Seeing him smile at me was one of my greatest pleasures. In fact, everything he did gave me joy. I would focus on every movement and facial expression David made, taking mental snap shots in my mind. Every moment was precious and I didn't want to miss a thing.

Suddenly those trivial things in life that I used to take so seriously— David spitting up on our new sofa, losing one of my diamond earrings, breaking a piece of our wedding crystal—were now insignificant.

Nothing mattered—just my life. I was beginning to look at the world differently because the world was now looking differently at me. I was undergoing a transformation—a new me. I liked the new me! Finally I was able to appreciate *everything*, and it was wonderful. I felt sad for not having discovered this sooner. I found beauty in and was enamored with everything I saw, heard, touched and smelled. For the first time in my life I truly felt alive!

Days later, as though ambushed from behind, my mind would automatically switch back to all of the fearful thoughts and situations I had created. I'd begin to panic and cry. When this would happen, I'd go to our bedroom and brood. I made a conscious effort not to allow myself to feel depressed, or mope around the house—that was not my character. I was always a cheerful person who would find pleasure in trying to raise the spirits of others who were feeling down. Yet, I was unsuccessful in helping myself.

In an attempt to keep my spirits up, I sought comfort from my family, relatives and friends—mainly from my dear friend Kathryn.

Kathryn and I worked for the same company for over ten years. She's a very knowledgeable and spiritual woman who's always been like a mother to me. I felt comfortable confiding in her because I knew I could trust her, and I always valued her wisdom. She was instrumental in assisting me through the grieving process after I lost my dad. She helped me cope and taught me how to accept things that I could not change. She bases her life on the philosophy that, *"everything is as it should be."* I chose to adopt her philosophy and not question the things I cannot change and the unknown—just accept them. It wasn't easy at first. In fact it was several months before I realized how right she was. Kathryn had been a cancer survivor for four years, so she knew firsthand the type of fear I was dealing with. I figured, if it worked for her perhaps it could work for me, too. I had nothing to lose and everything to gain.

Kathryn would call me two times a day, once in the morning and once in the evening just to make sure I was doing well. She also made herself available to me and encouraged me to call her any time of the day or night. Sometimes, I'd call her in a panic and she'd get me back on track. I can remember one conversation we had where I was asking her a series of "what if" questions. Questions, which to me where important and ought to be addressed. After all, I needed answers!

"What if I have to have chemotherapy? What if I need a mastectomy? What if I have a reoccurrence? What if I develop cancer in the other breast?" These were a few of the short-term things I feared most.

Kathryn advised me not to play the "what if" game and said I would only drive myself crazy in the process. And, she was right. Focusing on negative thoughts generated fear—fear that I couldn't afford to waste my energy on. Fear that was beginning to eat up every bit of energy that I needed to take care of myself and my family.

She'd always tell me not to worry about things that hadn't happened because chances are, they mostly likely wouldn't. "It isn't time to worry," she would say. Kathryn gave me an analogy that I could relate to just to make her point clear. It was about a new born baby.

"Nancy, you're a young new mother with a beautiful baby boy. Are you going to start worrying *now* about what will happen if he breaks his arm or leg? Are you going to start worrying *now* if he chooses not to go to college?" It finally hit home—I was worrying about things before it was time.

Cancer had become an all-consuming obsession for me. Sometimes I'd go out to our front porch to sit and think. The more I would think about where my life could be headed, the more depressed I became. I would just cry. I'd try to reflect back on my conversations with Kathryn and force my thoughts to turn around. But my fears began to invade again. I'd go in the house and back to our bedroom where I felt safe to be alone with my fears and anxieties.

Throughout the day I'd get several telephone calls. The telephone became my number one support vehicle. I'd get calls from my husband, my brother and sister, friends and relatives.

One day I received a phone call that led to another call that changed my life. It was from my cousin Leslie who lived in Wisconsin. Leslie and I grew up together and have always been close. She called to find out how I was feeling and could tell that I'd been crying. She tried her best to console me. During that conversation, she suggested that I call Father Yeprem Kelegian, the priest from Racine, Wisconsin, who officiated over our wedding and my dad's funeral. He was a wonderful man who provided me with the spiritual support I was lacking and so desperately needed.

I called Father Yeprem at St. Mesrob Armenian Church in Racine. Thank God (pun intended!) he was there to answer my desperate cry for help. He said a prayer for me over the phone. He also told me that he would put me on his silent prayer list during church services and would continue to pray for me daily.

I told him that after my dad passed away, I found it difficult to pray to God like I used to. I was angry at God for taking my dad away. Father Yeprem said, "God is a jealous God and He wants you on His side. You can still talk to Him when you're angry." Father Yeprem was right. When I hung up the phone I decided that I was going to have a one-on-one conversation with God.

Alone in our bedroom with the door closed, I laid on our bed and looked up at the ceiling. I shut my eyes as I poured my heart out to God.

God, you are my Father and I am your daughter. I will not question why this is happening to me. All I ask is that You give me the inner power and strength to accept the outcome, if this is Your will. This problem is too big for me to handle and I need to put my health in Your hands. Here it is Lord, I am now turning over this problem to You. Please take away this heavy burden I am carrying and provide me with peace of mind so I can at least sleep through the night and get through the crucial days that lie ahead. Lord, I know that I have failed to turn to You as I have in the past, but I'm turning to You now. I know You can forgive me for that Almighty God.

Why did You take my dad away from me? Why? Why didn't you answer my prayers? You made me very angry and now I feel like a hypocrite asking for Your help. Please God, I have a wonderful husband and a beautiful son that You blessed me with. I beg of You, do not let my life be limited. My family is counting on me just as I am counting on You. I love You God, and I love you too Daddy. Daddy, if you can hear me please be my guardian angel and watch over me and protect me like you did here on Earth. Again, Lord, I ask of You in Jesus' name to provide me with inner peace and give me the strength to accept and deal with whatever comes my way.

With my eyes still closed I began singing several verses of the biblical hymn, *"He's Got the Whole World in His Hands."* As I opened my eyes, suddenly I knew the Lord heard my call for help. I felt an inner peace that was inexplicable. I wondered if I was having a religious experience as I felt a tranquillity come over me. I closed my eyes again, as I didn't want this sense of serenity to leave my body.

I truly believed that when I turned my problems over to God he would take care of me and provide me with the strength I needed—not only to make it through these next several days of waiting for my biopsy results, but forever.

I believed that God was overjoyed that I had restored my faith in Him and wanted me to know that He heard my words. I was now operating from a new position of peace, happiness and confidence that I'd never before experienced. I praised my Almighty God and immediately got down on my knees to give thanks.

After the experience I called Father Yeprem to tell him about my revelation. I felt that I could see him smiling over the phone. He was so happy that I turned to God. He reinforced the fact that God cares and God listens. I thanked him again for his advice, and he said he would continue to pray for me. I told him that my mom was unaware of the situation at this point and that I would be telling her when she arrived. He asked that I keep him abreast of the test results, and I said that I would.

When I hung up the phone I immediately called my cousin Leslie to thank her for her suggestion. I began telling her what I had just experienced. She said she could tell from my voice that I had gone through a wonderful change.

When Randy came home from work, I gave him a big hug and told him how I spent the afternoon talking to Father Yeprem and God. I shared how much better I felt now that I'd turned everything over to God. I know Randy felt better too—it had been a long time since he'd seen me smile.

That night, my brother Tod came over. He was on his way to the airport to get our mom, who was coming to visit for the Thanksgiving holidays. Since Tod had an extra bedroom in his house, Mom would stay there.

"Are you ready to tell Mom about the cancer," he asked with concern. "Yes. I'm prepared—don't worry. Perhaps it would be best if you bring her directly here from the airport. Besides, I know she'll want to see David right away. Then once David is in bed for the night, Randy, you, and I can all sit down in the living room and I can tell to her. I really want you to be here when I tell her—she may need your support." "I think you're right," he said as he opened the door to leave for the airport. "I'll see you in about an hour."

I was very excited for my mom to see David. I loved the way she would smile and laugh when she was around him. Besides, I was anxious for her to see all of the changes in David since her last visit.

My mom arrived around eight o'clock, looking as beautiful as ever. She always looked at least 15 years younger than her true age. I always felt that she was too young to be a widow because she had so much life left to live—but don't we all. She's a fashionable woman who loves to accessorize with exotic jewelry, belts, and handbags that match her shoes. Everyone tells me what a nice dresser she is. And I couldn't agree more. In fact, when she'd come and visit, we'd often go shopping together and she'd help me pick out clothes and put together different outfits. My mom is an attractive woman, petite and very energetic. The phrase "shop 'til you drop" didn't apply to her—I'd drop long before she ever felt a need to stop and rest.

We exchanged our hugs and kisses and then I took her upstairs to see David, who was already in his crib. To our surprise, he was lying awake on his back looking straight up at his mobile. My mom leaned over and picked him up, smiling ear to ear.

"Just look at him!" she exclaimed. "He's gotten so big. I just love this little baby." She held him tightly and told me how blessed we were to have such a darling little boy. I could tell she wanted to play the goo-goo-gaah-gaah type of baby games that grandmothers play with their grandchildren, but didn't want to disturb his rest. "I'll have all day tomorrow to play with him, so I can wait," she said.

Watching my mom interact with David only made me wish that my dad were alive to share in the joy. My mom would always tell me how crazy my dad would have been over David—he adored children. That made me feel sadder than ever. To comfort me, my mom would say that my dad knows all about David and he can see him. Even if it were true, it still wasn't enough for me. I wanted to *see* my dad *see* our son—to love him, hold him, and play and interact with him like my mom did. She laid David back down in his crib and covered him with a blanket.

I was extremely anxious to tell my mom about the breast cancer. I had to get it off my chest (pun intended!).

"Let me tell you about my week, Mom," I began. "Last Tuesday I went to see my gynecologist and he found a lump in my breast—he thought it was a cyst or a clogged milk duct from breast feeding. Nonetheless, he had me go in for a mammogram." Her eyes widened, as she continued to listen to me without interrupting. "I had the mammogram on Wednesday. Thursday I went to see a breast specialist, and yesterday I had the lump removed." I pulled down the collar of my shirt and revealed my bandage to her. "Mom," I said in a strong voice, "I have breast cancer." I was amazed at how simple it was for me to tell her—and to tell her without shedding a tear. Then I felt much better just knowing that she knew, because I needed her motherly love and support. Her face dropped, as she tried to keep her composure. "How can this be? You're so young and we have no family history of breast cancer. Are you sure?" she asked.

"Yes, Mom. I have to wait until Tuesday before I get the pathology report," I said. "Mom, I wanted to tell you sooner but I didn't want you to worry over this and dwell on it your entire flight out here. I hope you can understand. Although I'm sure you won't sleep well tonight," I chuckled.

"You poor Honey—I wish I would have known," she reached out and gave me the biggest hug and kiss. I could tell she was overwhelmed and probably needed a hug from me as much as I needed one from her. A face which was so happy as she was holding our son just minutes ago now showed fear and concern. I felt responsible, and it broke my heart to cause her pain.

I wanted to spare her as much detail as possible until she was over the initial shock. Tod suggested that they go back to his house and unpack her things. When they left, I wondered what thoughts were going through her mind. How was she going to handle this? Did she start crying the minute she set foot out our door? This was supposed to be her Thanksgiving vacation, and now I'd taken the joy out of it.

Randy was very proud of how composed I had been when I told my mom. Things could have been a whole lot different had I been crying and carrying on.

The next day was Sunday—only two more days until I would get the results of the biopsy. I called my mom in the morning and asked her how she was. She told me she had a little difficulty sleeping and had been up since 4 a.m., waiting for a reasonable time to call her sisters and tell them about me. Who else could she turn to but her sisters? Her husband was gone, which made it even more difficult for her.

"How did they react?" I inquired.

"Well, they were all shocked and said they would pray for you. Your Aunt Catherine started to cry and felt just terrible. Aunt Catherine and I are very close—I think she adores me as much as I adore her. She's one of the most good-hearted people I know—truly angelic and a wonderful human being.

"I suppose everyone's going to feel bad Mom, and it hurts me to know that. I'm sorry to cause anyone any pain," I said, "but this is something I had no control over." "Well Honey, when people love you and care about you, they can't help but feel bad when bad things happen to you," she said compassionately.

After our conversation, I realized that I didn't want anyone to feel sorry for me or pity me in any way. That type of reaction would only make me feel like I was succumbing. If people were going to talk about me, I wanted to give them something positive to talk about. I wanted them to admire me for my strength and courage—not think of me as wallowing in the negatives of having developed the disease. I tried my hardest to project an upbeat and positive attitude.

The next few days I tried to keep busy doing things with my mom.

Actually, I think it was therapeutic for both of us. We'd go shopping, take David on stroller rides, feed the ducks at the park, and go out to lunch and just talk.

One day while we were having lunch my mom asked me if I was putting on an act. "An act?" I questioned. "Yes. You're acting as if nothing is wrong. Are you trying to be strong around me so I won't worry? I'm your mother, you can talk to me about anything."

"I know I can Mom, but I'm really okay. I called Father Yeprem and he helped me with great spiritual support."

"You mean Father Yeprem knows? I'm so glad you talked to him."

"So am I. The conversation I had with him led me to have a conversation with God. The experience changed my life forever. I'm not carrying the burden any more. God is. He will give me the strength I need to get through this no matter what. I honestly believe that."

I shared the details of my experience with her and how I talked to Dad and asked him to be my guardian angel and watch over me like he did here on Earth.

"I know he is, Nancy. You and your dad had a very special relationship. You were the apple of his eye," she said.

That afternoon Mom offered to look after David so Randy and I could spend some time alone together. Randy decided to take me to a movie to get my mind focused on something else. He asked me what movie I'd like to see and I chose, *The Mirror has Two Faces*, starring Barbra Streisand and Jeff Bridges.

It was my first time out in public after my operation. I can remember sitting down in the crowded theater and feeling so alone and singled out. I felt different. No one here knows I have breast cancer, I thought. No one cares. It seemed like everyone's lives remain unchanged—except mine.

I can't say that I remember much about the movie. I just remember seeing Barbra Streisand in several sexy low-cut dresses, which made matters worse. I kept wondering if I was going to lose my breast and if I'd ever feel whole and feminine again.

After the movie we took a short drive down to a quaint little city called San Juan Capistrano. On our way, I told Randy that I was probably the only one in the theater dealing with cancer. He turned to look at me and placed his hand on my thigh, "Nancy, everyone has problems at one time or another, you just don't know what they are." How true. Yet I couldn't help but wonder if their problems were as big as mine. I sensed that I was gradually beginning to lose my mental strength and I was returning to my *old* way of thinking, not remembering that everything is relative to everyone.

When we got to San Juan Capistrano, Randy spotted a few antique shops and asked if I wanted to go in. He knew how much I enjoyed shopping for antiques and finding special treasures. We strolled in and out of a few shops but I just couldn't get into it. Randy found this rather odd, because he knew I had such a strong passion for antiques, but he understood why.

"How about going to that department store up the street? Maybe you'll want something new instead," he said in a playful manner. We walked arm in arm down the street until we got to the store. I browsed, but nothing caught my eye. I felt strange. I felt different. I felt like I was alone in a crowd of people. I began to sweat and feel uneasy. Then I started to panic. I turned around to find Randy who was only a few feet away. I grabbed his arms and began hugging him tightly as I buried my face in his chest. I broke down and started crying hysterically.

"Randy," I cried, "I can't take this anymore! I'm so afraid. Why is this happening to me? I was doing so well and being so strong until now."

"You're allowed to get upset, Nancy." He held me tight and wiped away my tears. "It's going to be okay," he said trying to reassure me. "You're going to be fine." He guided me outside of the store to get some fresh air. We slowly walked toward the car.

"I wanna go home." I said. "I'm wiped out!"

When we arrived home, my mother greeted us. She said she had just put David down for his nap, and that he had been a very good boy.

That's one thing I must say: God blessed us with a very easy baby. He'd rarely fuss, even when we'd put him down for his naps. I never knew he was teething until a tooth came in—that's how easy he was. I couldn't imagine having a difficult baby on top of everything else I was going through.

My mom could sense that I was not myself. That's one thing about mothers—they can immediately tell when something's wrong with their children. I told my mom I was tired and was going up to our bedroom to rest. I'm sure she asked Randy if we had a nice time together, and whether or not we enjoyed the movie. My mom and Randy have a close mother-son-like relationship. I'm sure they leaned on one another, taking turns sharing feelings and providing support to each other. After all, they share a common ground—they both love me!

I wasn't able to rest—my head was spinning like a roulette wheel. I needed someone to comfort me so I called Kathryn. She was the only one (next to God) who I could talk to to help me get me out of my funk. God didn't talk—Kathryn did. She told me that it was okay for me to have these feelings. "If you didn't have these feelings Nancy, you wouldn't be normal." She would always tell me to *be happy: act as if, and then you will become.* Kathryn was one of the first people I would call whenever I'd get in the crisis mode. I felt as though she was my personal trainer, getting my mind in shape to win the "Gold Mental" Olympics. She tried training me to go to a special place in my mind—a place where I could visualize having a lot of fun.

"Go to Disneyland," she'd say. "You can only think of one thing at a time, so why not think about Disneyland."

"I hear it's suppose to be the happiest place on earth," I'd say facetiously. We both started laughing.

I admire Kathryn for her inner strength. She was like an iron butterfly—strong on the inside and graceful on the outside. I wanted to be able to think like her and would tell her that all of the time.

"I didn't use to be like this Nancy. It took years and years of practice. I evolved, and so will you. You're handling this beautifully and are very receptive to letting me help you. Most people would just wallow in their sorrows, but not you. We'll get through this," she said. It made me feel so good when she'd say those words—"We'll get through this." The fact that she used the word "we'll" made me feel as though she was embracing my problems and I wasn't facing them alone. Kathryn and I would talk at length several times a day. She would never allow me to hang up the phone until I felt better emotionally. Everyone should have a Kathryn in his or her life—especially when going through a crisis such as this. People need people.

Monday came and Monday went. It seemed as though I was talking on the phone all day long. Friends and relatives were calling me constantly. It was so reassuring. Everyone I talked to said they would pray for me. Some people went as far as putting me on prayer lists and lighting candles for me during their church services. All of this helped give me the comfort that I needed. It made me feel good to know that people cared and wanted to help.

One of my mom's friends said that she called a nationwide prayer chain to have prayers said for me 24 hours a day, seven days a week, for 30 consecutive days. I was thankful that she gave me the phone number because I called it during one of my many hours of desperation and put myself on the prayer chain too! It made me feel spiritually enriched— knowing that *I* was contributing to my own cause. It also gave me a sense of having *some* control over my destiny.

I was also very fortunate to have a dear friend in the medical field who served as another spiritual guide. Dr. Debbie, as I refer to her, is a family practice physician at a nearby healthcare facility. Randy introduced me to Debbie and Matt, now her husband, when we first started dating. Matt and Randy were fraternity brothers at Ohio State University and both ended up living in Southern California. On weekends, and sometimes during the week, we'd all get together and go out to dinner, the movies, sporting events, or other activities. They were the couple that we did the most with. I was blessed to have Debbie as my friend because I could talk to her not only as my friend, but as a woman and a doctor too. She was able to put the medical jargon in to layman's terms for me. Many times I would wake up in the middle of the night with scary thoughts and questions that would keep me from falling back to sleep. Whenever this would happen, I'd get out of bed and jot them down on a piece of paper—this helped me clear my head and prevented the thought from reoccurring. Then whenever Debbie would call to see how I was doing, I'd pull out my list of questions and read them to her one by one. She was more than happy to address them for me, which helped to put my mind at ease. As busy as she was, she always made time for me.

4

I woke up feeling extremely anxious, but was relieved that Tuesday was finally here, and by two o'clock that afternoon the waiting would be over. I would have answers. Good or bad, I needed to know. The morning hours seemed endless. The suspense of the unknown began to gnaw at me. I realized I needed God's help to jump-start my day. Once again I asked Him to give me strength to accept the outcome—even if it meant losing my breast and/or undergoing chemotherapy.

To break up the day, my mom and I decided to go out to a Chinese restaurant for lunch. Toward the end of our meal, my mom put her hand over mine and said, "Honey, I'm so proud of you. You're so strong. I don't think I could be as strong as you." It made me feel good to hear her say that, because that's how I wanted to be perceived—not only by my mother, but by everyone who knew I had breast cancer.

"Oh, yes you could. If you put everything in God's hands you can get through anything," I said. "I want you to know I can handle this, Mom. I'm prepared to do whatever it takes—even if it means losing a breast! It's a small price to pay for my life and I want to live a long one so I can be here for Randy and David," I said.

Just then our waitress brought us the bill, along with two fortune cookies. I looked at my mom and asked, "Which cookie do you want?"

"You choose first," she said sliding the tray of cookies to me.

"I'll take this one—the one closest to me," I said opening up the wrapper. I broke the cookie in half and pulled out the little slip of paper tucked inside containing my fortune.

"What does it say?" my mom asked curiously.

"It says, "Put up with small annoyances to gain great results.""

"Well, isn't that appropriate?"

"It sure is. Maybe this is a sign that everything's going to be okay!" I said with a smile. My mom gave me a hug, and we walked out to the car.

Trying to fight my feelings of anxiety, I turned on the car stereo and made small-talk with my mom until we arrived at the breast center.

I *really* began to feel nervous as we started walking from the parking lot to Dr. Baick's office. I had more than butterflies in my stomach, I had bats!

"Mom," I said. "Will you come in to the exam room with me and Randy to hear the results? I don't want you sitting out here alone wondering what the outcome is."

"Of course I will, Honey. I'm just as anxious to hear what the doctor has to say."

Randy was to meet us at Dr. Baick's office shortly before my appointment. I was grateful that he was able to arrange his work schedule to be with me.

The receptionist greeted us as I signed in. She told us to have a seat and said Dr. Baick had two patients to see before me. I couldn't help but notice the two other women in the waiting room who appeared to be in their early to mid-60s'. I'm sure both of them assumed that I was accompanying my mother to see *her* doctor instead of the other way around—it seemed only logical based on our ages. Both of the women appeared to be undergoing chemotherapy treatment and looked rather frail. One woman was wearing a black turban to cover her hair loss; the other was wearing a wig.

The palms of my hands began to sweat as I wondered if I'd be facing a similar experience. My anxiety level peaked. I tried to remind myself that there are several types of breast cancers, and not all women undergo the same type of treatment for the disease.

I picked up a magazine hoping that reading would help me relax. I found myself unable to concentrate or comprehend what I was reading, so I resorted to looking at the pictures.

I longed for Randy to arrive—he always gave me the security that I needed, even without saying a word. About 15 minutes later, Randy walked in looking as handsome as ever in his suit and tie. He smiled as he sat down next to me and interlocked his fingers with mine. I gazed into his brown eyes thinking how lucky I am to have such a wonderful husband whose love for me is endless.

"How are you holding up?" he asked.

"As well as can be expected," I replied. I pulled out the fortune from my wallet and showed it to him.

He read it with a smile and said, "Now that's something positive."

"I hope so," I said. "We'll soon find out."

We waited another 15 minutes before my name was finally called.

The three of us were escorted down the hall to the first examination room on the right where we impatiently waited for Dr. Baick behind the closed door.

I kept staring at the door anxiously waiting for it to open. In the background, we could hear Dr. Baick talking to his nurse. If I wasn't forced to follow protocol, I would have yanked the door open, popped my head out of the exam room and shouted, "Dr. Baick, tell me if my cancer is invasive or non-invasive?!" That was the *main* question I needed to have answered, as it would determine whether or not I would need to have a mastectomy and/or undergo chemotherapy treatment. We were all hoping that when Dr. Baick came in to deliver my results, we would hear the word "non-invasive," meaning the cancer didn't travel and multiply through the lymphatic system and I wouldn't need chemotherapy.

The suspense of finding out the results was unbearable. I'd waited long enough—I needed to know NOW. Suddenly, I heard my file being pulled from the folder holder on the opposite side of the door. The door opened. Dr. Baick walked in with the file in his hands and laid it on the counter. I was so relieved to finally see him and hear the report. I introduced Dr. Baick to my mother before he proceeded.

"Fortunately, the cancer was detected early," he said. "We rank cancers in terms of stages—Stage 1 is an early stage and Stage 4 is the latest. Your cancer is Stage 1, and very aggressive. The lump measured 1.1 centimeters in size, about this big," he said showing me his pinkie fingernail. "The type of cancer you have is called *ductal carcinoma in situ*—it's a non-invasive cancer that arises in the ducts of the breast and hasn't spread past the edges of the tumor." I listened attentively to every word he spoke trying only to find the positives.

When I heard the word "non-invasive" I knew it meant I didn't need to have a mastectomy and/or undergo chemotherapy. I started crying tears of joy and felt a major sense of relief. I could see that Randy and my mother were relieved too. Nonetheless, I needed Dr. Baick's confirmation.

"Non-invasive means I don't need to have a mastectomy and/or chemotherapy, right?"

"There is a very slight chance that you may need to have chemotherapy as one microscopic cell was detected outside the margin block of tissue that was removed," he explained. I began feeling uneasy all over again.

"How slight is slight?" I asked nervously. "Only a three percent chance," he replied.

"I don't think I need to be overly concerned with odds like that—I'm just thankful that it's non-invasive. How will you determine the final outcome?" I asked.

"We'll have to perform another surgery to remove some of your lymph nodes just to ensure that the cancer has not spread to your lymphatic system—it's called an axillary node dissection."

I threw my upper torso over the examination table with my hands cupped over my forehead, "Oh, no, not another operation!" I exclaimed.

"Don't worry, this is just a precautionary procedure. Alice will explain the procedure to you and set up the surgery date," he said.

We were led down the hall to another examination room where Alice was waiting for us. I introduced her to my mother and thanked her for all of her support.

"You're very fortunate," she said. Many young women aren't as lucky as you. They are faced with having to undergo chemotherapy, a mastectomy, and sometimes both."

This reconfirmed my belief in God. I knew He had heard my cry for help and had listened to all of the prayers people had been saying for me. Regardless of what *I* wanted, God had the final word. God spared my life, and I am forever grateful unto Him.

Alice said the operation would involve a recovery process of approximately six weeks. "Dr. Baick will make an incision in your axillary gland, right about here," she said pointing inside my underarm. "He'll remove anywhere from 12 to 20 lymph nodes to get an adequate sampling. During surgery, a drain will be inserted along your right side. It looks like this," she said holding up a clear long tube. Your body will drain the fluid through the tube and it will collect in here," she said pointing to what looked like a grenade attached to the end of the tube.

"How long will the drain have to stay in?" I asked, dreading the entire procedure.

"Oh, a week to ten days. You'll have to empty the fluid in your drain a few times a day and record the amount of cc's," she pointed to a measuring cup with a cc scale on it. "The hospital will give you one so you can measure and record the fluid you're draining." I continued to listen closely as she picked up a small rectangular metal box with a few buttons on it. "You'll also be going home with a gadget like this. It's called a PCA which stands for patient controlled analgesia. This machine will allow you to administer a controlled amount of morphine into your system to relieve any pain you may have. All you have to do is press this," she said pointing to the small black button.

"Will I be spending the night in the hospital?" I asked.

"No, this is an outpatient surgery. However, you will have a visiting nurse come to your home the following day to make sure you're doing alright. Let me go see when we scheduled the surgery," she said as she left the room.

"It sounds like a lot of monkey business to me," I said to my mom and Randy.

"It does sound rather complicated," my mom said. "Honey, if you'd like, I can extend my stay and help you out. I think you're going to need it," she said warmheartedly.

"That would be great. I really want you to be here, Mom," I said with tears in my eyes.

When Alice re-entered the room she told me that my surgery date was scheduled for Monday morning, December 2. She provided me with a list of instructions and told me not to eat after midnight the night before the operation.

"Do you have any questions?" she asked.

"No, but I'm sure I'll have plenty after the operation," I said as we got up to leave the room.

"Well, have a wonderful Thanksgiving and don't worry about anything else. Just enjoy the time with your family."

"I will Alice, you too," I said.

"We really have a lot to be thankful for this Thanksgiving," Randy said.

"We sure do," my mom chimed in.

"Let's go—I have a lot of phone calls to make. Everyone's waiting to hear my news," I said.

When we got home I called Laura, my friend from work. I shared with her the outcome of my appointment. "That's such great news, Nancy. Don't even worry about the three percent chance that it's invasive. Look at it as a 97 percent chance that it's not," she said. She had a valid point. Laura had her own special way of making me feel better. "I'll be sure to tell Marcia, Maria, and the others in our department. Everyone's been asking about you."

"Thanks Laura. Tell them I'm doing fine. I'll keep in touch."

The entire evening I was on the telephone sharing the news with almost everyone I knew, telling them that my cancer was non-invasive. It got to the point where I was tired of repeating the same story—plus, I needed time to be with my family and just relax. I asked a few of my relatives and friends to serve as point persons and disseminate my health report to others in our social circle. That helped a great deal.

It was finally time to tell my three best friends, Mary, Edna, and Sandi. I deliberately spared telling them about my breast cancer diagnosis until I had more facts. I knew it would be devastating, but they all needed to know.

Mary and I had been friends since seventh grade. We attended junior high, high school and college together. We were like sisters. Some people say a friendship can be ruined by living together, but not ours. Having Mary as my roommate solidified our friendship. We shared a dorm room together in the early 1980's at the University of Wisconsin-Milwaukee. It was there that Mary and I met Edna and Sandi and decided to share our first apartment together off campus. Mary and I were roommates for four years; two of which were with Edna and one with Sandi.

After college, I was the first one to move away. My brother Tod suggested I seek employment in Southern California and move near him, so I did. Within one week I landed my first professional job as an account coordinator at an advertising agency, and decided to make California my new home. It was sad leaving my family and friends, but I felt a need to move to where the job opportunities were.

Edna was the first one of us to get married. She met her husband Tim in Spain—both were studying Spanish abroad for a semester. Tim is from Memphis, Tennessee, so a few months after Edna graduated, they were married and she moved there.

In 1992, Mary and I both met our soul mates. She met George shortly before I met Randy—our lives were beginning to parallel. She married George the following year and moved to Rantoul, Illinois.

Sandi's still searching for her soul mate. She moved to Los Angeles shortly after she graduated to pursue a career in the film industry. It's nice having at least one of my best friends living nearby. Sandi is a very unique individual. She's the type of person who will say and do strange things to make people laugh. I decided to call her first and tell her what had been going on. When I told her I was diagnosed with breast cancer, she was speechless and didn't know what to say except, "I'll pray for you."

I knew Mary was most likely to take the news the hardest as we had such a long history together. Besides, we lost our fathers to cancer within two months of each other. My dad passed away first. We mourned the loss of our fathers and grieved openly to each other for months over the phone. Our losses were similar—our fathers were our heroes and we were daddies' girls. Our parents had developed a closeness through our friendship which only multiplied the sorrows. I knew Mary would get emotional and cry if I told her I had breast cancer. When family and friends would cry for me (as sympathetic as they were), I felt as though they thought I was going to die—and perhaps that's what they actually thought! I learned that many people are not as educated on this disease as I assumed they would be. In fact, I didn't know much about breast cancer until I developed it. Nonetheless, subjecting myself to emotional people had a negative impact on my ability to stay positive.

I asked Sandi to do me the favor of telling Mary and Edna, as I was too mentally exhausted to tell two more friends. She agreed to tell them for me. Within minutes of hearing the news, Mary called. I sensed she was holding back her tears, "What the heck is going on?" she asked. I explained everything to her from the beginning and told her that I didn't have the heart to tell her myself because she had been through enough with her dad.

"Nancy, you know I'm always here for you. Don't let things like that stand in your way. I'm going to light a candle for you in church on Sunday," she said.

"Thanks Mary. I'll be fine," I said.

Just then I received a call-waiting beep on my phone. It was Edna.

"Hi, Edna. I just got off the phone with Mary."

"I just heard the news from Sandi, are you okay?" she asked with concern.

"Yes, but I've been living a nightmare this past week," I said.

Once again, I went on to explain. She, too, said she'd pray for me and put me on a prayer list at her church. That warmed my heart.

The days leading up to my second operation were peaceful and stress-free, unlike the previous week. Although I had to undergo another operation, I felt confident that the cancer hadn't spread into my lymph nodes. The odds of that happening were extremely low. I believed God, together with my guardian angel (my dad), had carried me to safety and would continue watching over me.

I finally began to feel as though there was some semblance to my life again—the waiting was over! I felt a massive sense of relief knowing that I didn't have to have a mastectomy and more than likely wouldn't have to undergo chemotherapy either.

Almost every morning, I'd go on long walks by myself and give thanks to God for having spared my life. I'd make up songs as I strolled through my neighborhood singing aloud, *"I'm feelin' fine. Everything's gonna be all right. God's on my side. He'll make it right."*

While on these walks, I often thought how different my situation could have been had the lump gone undetected. Since I never practiced self-breast exams in the past, the lump could have grown much, much larger before I ever discovered it. The cancer, as aggressive as it was, could have multiplied and eventually traveled into lymph nodes. Then where would I be? The thought of my life being cut short was horrifying.

Facing my own mortality caused me to truly appreciate life and everything surrounding me. Having life and experiencing life is something that should not be taken for granted. Every moment is precious; yet many of us fail to realize it (myself included), until something tragic strikes… then all of a sudden, we wake up and realize that we've been living our lives entirely wrong! Every day is a gift—that's why it's call the *present*.

Everything I once took for granted had now come to mean so much, for now I was looking at the world through new eyes. I remembered reading about cancer survivors who would say that getting cancer was one of the best things that could have happened to them. It never made any sense to me then, but it certainly does now.

Cancer forces one to value life's moments—not things. It makes one realize just how precious life *really* is. It makes one stop and think about what's *really* important and helps one set new priorities. Cancer also forces a person to think about things that he or she should have done but never did—whether it's mending a lost relationship, spending more time with the family, or simply saying, "I love you."

I pondered on what caused me to get this disease in the first place. Was it the stress from my father's death? Was it because I didn't eat enough fruits and vegetables? Was it because I ate too much red meat and didn't exercise enough? I tried not to drive myself crazy with these questions, but they did enter my mind. I just wanted to know what *I* did to cause it, or what *I* could have done to prevent it. I felt responsible somehow.

I read many books, talked to several medical doctors and cancer specialists, yet no one knew the answer. I actually found solace in knowing that no one had the answers. Why? Because if I knew what caused breast cancer, and somehow I could have prevented it, I would have spent more time and energy wishing I hadn't done what I did to get it. In other words, if I were told that my cancer was caused because I ate too many yellow jellybeans, I would have spent the majority of my life regretting the fact that I ate too many yellow jellybeans! I'd wallow in self-blame.

The cause of cancer remains a mystery. There are no forewarnings. Cancer plays no favorites. It lays dormant then gradually decides to creep into the lives of young and old. Manifesting, mutating, multiplying, and surging throughout the body in silent destruction.

Major medical strides have already been made since my diagnosis. And I'm hopeful that there will be a cure for this disease in my lifetime. Not only for breast cancer, but cancer in general. If not in my lifetime, I hope in David's.

*   *   *   *   *   *   *   *   *   *

Our family celebrated Thanksgiving at my brother's house with my mother that year. The Thanksgiving holiday suddenly took on a new meaning for our family as we celebrated and gave thanks for all of God's gifts—including my victory over cancer.

Before I knew it, the day of my axillary node dissection had arrived. Randy took the day off from work and drove me to the hospital. My mom came too, for moral support. I was anxious to have the operation, get the results, and resume a *normal* life. It had been weeks since I felt any type of normalcy! I so badly wanted to enjoy being a new mom and do fun things as a family with my husband and son.

I was slightly nervous about undergoing this operation. It sounded like it was going to be a long recovery process—especially since I had to be away from work for six weeks.

When I awoke from the operation, I was left in the recovery room for approximately 45 minutes. I still felt heavily sedated. It was much more difficult waking up after this operation than it was from the lumpectomy.

I noticed the drains hanging on my right side along with my controlled morphine device. Over my bandages was a bra-like garment that zipped up the front. It had heavy-duty adjustable Velcro straps designed to keep my gauze and drains in place. The nurses helped me get dressed, and put me in a wheel chair.

"Your husband and your mother are going to bring the car around," said one of nurses as she wheeled me outside. The sun was extremely bright; I put my head down and closed my eyes. I just wanted to go home and sleep.

Randy got out of the car and assisted the nurse in seating me in the car. I have no memory of the ride home, as I must have slept the entire way. When we got home, Randy escorted me up the stairs to our bedroom where I rested the majority of the day and evening. I experienced some discomfort while sleeping, mainly due to all of the tubes that were attached to me. I had no choice but to sleep on my back. I was given Vicodin, a painkiller, to take every four to six hours, as well as Keflex, an antibiotic to prevent infections.

The visiting nurse came to our house the next morning. I was glad to see her because I was confused and overwhelmed about what to do with all of the apparatus that was hanging from my side. I remembered Alice showing me all of these things and explaining them to me, yet somehow having all of the tubes dangling from my right side along with the hand-held morphine device caused my mind to go blank.

Fortunately, the nurse went over everything with me again, including measuring and logging the amount of fluid I was draining. She also explained how important it was for me to be careful of my right arm and not to injure it in any way for the rest of my life.

"Even a small paper cut or doing gardening work can be dangerous now because you don't have the lymph nodes to fight off infection. If you do get cut, make sure you clean the area really well with hydrogen peroxide. You want to avoid infection at all costs because you could be susceptible to a condition called lymphedema."

"What's that?" I asked.

"Lymphedema is a swelling of the arm or hand caused by excess fluid that collects after lymph nodes and vessels are removed. Going forward, you should never allow anyone to take your blood pressure on your right arm because it cuts off your circulation. You really need to be protective of this arm," she said.

The following day I had an appointment to see Dr. Baick for the postoperative visit. He said I was doing well and should call him on Friday for the results of the axillary node biopsy. He removed the handheld morphine device, which gave me the freedom of not having to carry it around anymore. I think I only used the morphine once—mainly out of curiosity—not pain. I just wanted to push the button (like a little kid) to see what it would do, only to discover that it just made a lot of noise! Dr. Baick said the drain would more than likely be removed next week.

The most inconvenient part of this operation was not being able to take a shower or shave under my arms. I had to take sponge baths and wash my hair over the kitchen sink for two weeks. Since I was unable to reach my head with two hands, my mom and Randy would take turns washing my hair for me.

On Friday, Earlene, a registered nurse from Dr. Baick's office, called to tell me that the pathology report came back and I was fine! She said I had 17 lymph nodes removed, all of which were negative. I was now cancer-free!

"I knew you would want to know this, so I called you just as soon as the report hit my desk. I'm glad that everything's turning out well for you, Nancy," she said.

"Thanks Earlene," I said with a huge smile on my face. I hung up the phone and raced down the stairs to tell my mother who was feeding David, "Mom! Mom!" I cried.

"What Honey, what's wrong?" she asked.

"Nothing's wrong! All of my lymph nodes are cancer-free! All 17 of 'em!"

"Oh that's wonderful—I knew they would be," she said giving me a big hug.

"I knew they would be too, but it's always nice to have that confirmation!" I looked at David and said, "Your mama's gonna be okay. I love you so much," I said kissing him on the top of his head.

I made a few phone calls to various people to let them know that I was officially cancer-free.

When I called Marcia, my director at work, she was thrilled to hear the good news, and said she would tell the others in our department.

"Hurry back. We miss you around here. Besides, I have a lot of work for you to do," she said jokingly.

I was anxious to get back to work to see my friends and have some normalcy restored to my life. Unfortunately, I wasn't fully recovered yet. I still had approximately five more weeks before Dr. Baick would release me.

Every day I'd continue to measure and log the fluid my body was draining. And, every day the amount of fluid began to lessen and lessen. This confirmed that the drain would be removed at my next office visit, just as Dr. Baick had said.

Sure enough, at the next office visit the drain was removed. I felt so free. Although I did not have full range of motion with my arm yet, I knew exercising it would be the next step in helping me regain its full use.

"Can I take showers now?" I asked hopefully.

"No, not yet. We have to wait for the drain holes on your right side to heal. Give it a few more days," Dr. Baick said. I hated having that restriction. I longed to take a shower more than anything!

Margo, one of Dr. Baick's Medical Assistants, showed me how to clean the area and position the gauze over the incision. She also gave me a list of exercises to begin doing at home. The first one was called "climbing the wall" which entailed standing an arms distance from the wall and walking my fingers up the wall as high as I could. The other exercise was called "making circles" which involved bending at the waist and letting my right arm hang. As it hung, I'd make little circles with my right arm gradually working up to making bigger circles. I did these exercises three to five times a day. They were quite easy, although a little uncomfortable to master at first. However, the more I exercised my arm, the more limber it became.

Christmas was just around the corner. I so badly wanted to attend our department Christmas party, which was to be held in a private room at a very fancy restaurant. My mom offered to baby-sit and felt it would be good for Randy and me to get dressed up, go out, and mingle with others. She had a good point, so we decided to go.

I was unsure as to how my co-workers would receive me. I knew they were very concerned about my health. I tried to put them at ease by making an effort to approach everyone and give them a Christmas hug. They were all very happy that I had attended and were glad to see that I was doing well.

Before dinner, Marcia made a toast, thanking everyone for their hard work and commitment. It warmed my heart when she included my name in the toast—thanking me for coming and wishing me good health.

Before long, arrangements of colorful flowers and beautiful plants were being delivered to our home. Our mailbox was overflowing with get-well cards.

Friends, neighbors, relatives and associates from work would come over to visit me on a regular basis. Pastor Tim McCalmont, from The Presbyterian Church of the Covenant in Costa Mesa, where Randy and I sometimes attended, also came to visit me. Although we never officially joined the church, Pastor Tim treated us as though we were members and had his congregation pray for me.

When Toni, one of the members from the church, found out I had breast cancer, she had contacted Pastor Tim and asked him to call me to see if I would mind if he gave Toni my telephone number. Toni took a special interest in my situation because she had developed breast cancer in her mid-20's, and has been a cancer survivor for over 25 years.

Toni truly has the Lord in her heart. She radiates love and happiness. She talked about her own experience with me and then began to pray for me over the phone. I closed my eyes as I listened to her ask God to heal me. Her prayers were so beautiful they made me cry; I know God heard her. I was getting stronger everyday.

I continued to exercise my arm and was able to notice an improvement in my range of motion. Dr. Baick noticed the improvement too, and said I was progressing nicely, which was encouraging to hear.

"So what's the next step?" I asked.

"Well, you'll be monitored closely, as all cancer patients are, for the next five years," he said. "You'll need to have a mammogram every year, and have blood drawn every three months for the first three years and then every six months years four and five. After five years, you'll need to be seen once a year."

It sounded like my life was going to be consumed with doctors' visits—but I had to do whatever it took to stay on top of this disease. I didn't mind being monitored so closely, in fact, it made me feel more comfortable. I knew that if something was ever found, it would be detected early—and that's always preferable.

"I can handle that," I said confidently. I thought that was all I needed to do. Unfortunately, it wasn't.

"I'd like Dr. Mahmood, one of our medical oncologists, to review your case. The receptionist will set up an appointment for you to have a consultation with him."

Since Dr. Mahmood was affiliated with Dr. Baick's staff, I felt comfortable going to see him, as I knew Dr. Baick only worked with the best.

That evening I called my friend Dr. Debbie and told her how I was referred to see a medical oncologist. She said that was not uncommon and helped me put together a list of questions to ask, many of which involved medical terms that I'd never heard of. She asked me to find out if my estrogen and progesterone receptors were positive or negative.

"What's that suppose to mean?" I asked.

She explained, "During pregnancy, your body produces many hormones. Some of the female hormones that are produced can cause some breast cancers to grow more. But if you don't have receptors for these hormones then we'll know there was no correlation between the hormones your body produced during pregnancy, and the breast cancer itself. Let's just hope your receptors are both negative," she said.

She also told me that cancer can be more aggressive in premenopausal women and slower growing in post-menopausal women. "That's why you're so lucky that it was detected early, as well as being non-invasive cancer. Many of my young patients aren't as lucky as you," she said.

I wanted to know everything I might expect. She mentioned something about a drug called "Tamoxifin". She said it was a drug used and tested for many years, which actually helped reduce the chance of reoccurrence. It is mainly used for women beyond menopause. However, she felt that the side effects could be more difficult for me to deal with than the actual benefit, and advised me to discuss it with the oncologist.

Later in the week, Randy and I went to see Dr. Mahmood. We both felt very comfortable with him, and were impressed with how thorough he was. He discussed my results with us in great detail, drawing pictures and diagrams to educate us even further.

"You are one lucky lady," he said. "Had you waited another three to six months you could have been faced with having a mastectomy and chemotherapy."

"How long do you think the cancer was inside my breast before it was detected?" I asked.

"Oh, I'd guess about three or four months," he said.

My mind reverted back to what had occurred at that time in my life. Since David was already five-months-old, that meant I most likely developed cancer just *after* he was born. Hence, the timing of his birth had a direct impact on the cancer being detected. Had I not become pregnant, my annual check-up with my gynecologist would have been almost a year later. It's ironic how *giving* life *saved* my life. I'm just thankful that my gynecologist, Dr. Kraus, was proactive and advised me to have a mammogram. He could have easily said, "come back in six months and we'll do a re-check." Had that been the case, I'd be facing a mastectomy and chemotherapy. Dr. Kraus is truly responsible for sav ing my life, and I later told him so.

"Were my progesterone and estrogen receptors positive or negative?" I asked, feeling sophisticated with the new medical terminology I had just learned from Dr. Debbie.

"They're both negative—your cancer had nothing to do with your pregnancy," he said confidently.

"Does that mean we can have more children?" my husband asked.

"Yes. That shouldn't be a problem. However, I am recommending that you undergo radiation therapy to the right breast. I suggest that you wait six months afterwards to give your body a rest before you try conceiving another baby," he said.

"We didn't want to start that soon anyway," I said. "We've decided to wait until our son is at least two years old," I said, evading the word radiation.

"Why are you recommending radiation?" Randy asked.

"It's a means to ensure that any remaining cancerous or pre-cancerous cells that surrounded the cancer site are destroyed. That way the body will continue producing only normal healthy cells," he said.

"What are the odds of reoccurrence?" I asked.

"Chances are extremely low. It's the opposite breast that you need to continue to watch. If you live to be 85 years old you'll have a 30 percent lifetime chance. That's 0.8 percent per year—that's pretty good," he said.

"That's less than a 1 percent chance per year Nancy, that's really good," said Randy. I felt comfortable knowing that, but I knew there would always be some fear in the back of my mind the older I'd become.

"In the event that you developed a reoccurrence after your radiation therapy, we'd have to perform a mastectomy as we cannot give you any more radiation treatments—you'll have received the maximum. Just hearing the word *mastectomy* made me cringe. I chose not to dwell on that portion of the conversation and immediately asked another question.

"Are you going to put me on the drug Tamoxifin?" I asked.

"No, I don't think you'll be a good candidate for that," he said.

Still thinking about the possibilities of a reoccurrence and a new occurrence, I said, "I hate to admit this Dr. Mahmood, but I'm not quite sure I know exactly how to do a breast exam," I said.

"You just need to be concerned with your left breast," he said. He showed me what to do and instructed me to feel as high up as my collarbone. "Make sure you really know your breast. Keep a mental note of what you feel and where you feel it. If there's anything—anything at all that feels strange to you, make an appointment to see Dr. Baick," he said.

"I'm going to refer you to see Dr. Ngo, our head radiologist. He'll be able to answer any questions you may have going forward. He's also affiliated with our medical staff. I'm going to close out your file because I don't think I'll need to see you again," he said.

I felt so good walking out of his office. The only thing that bothered me was his recommendation that I undergo radiation therapy. When we got home I shared the news with my mom—I told her how fortunate Dr. Mahmood said I was about having detected the cancer so early, and that had I waited another three to six months I'd be facing a mastectomy and chemotherapy.

"Thank God. I thank God everyday," she said hugging me tightly. "Mom, will you come to my radiation consultation next week?" Iasked. "I can have Clara baby-sit again."

"Of course I will, Sweetheart, you know that," she said.

It seemed like every time I received an important piece of news from my doctors, I would turn around and call my support circle of friends and family. I did my best to keep them abreast (pun intended!) of what was happening.

When I called Kathryn to tell her that my medical oncologist suggested I have radiation therapy, she offered to take the afternoon off from work and come with me. I was thrilled that she would do this for me. Since Kathryn had to undergo radiation when she was diagnosed with cancer, I figured she would be a good source of support in that regard, too. For some reason, I wasn't overly concerned about having to undergo radiation therapy, as this was the only means of destroying any surrounding cancer cells that may have been left behind. I knew we needed to take an aggressive approach, and radiation was it.

5

I was looking forward to having the radiation consultation with Dr. Ngo. I was calm and had no reservations about undergoing the necessary treatments—at least not yet. I was thrilled that Kathryn had offered to accompany me. It was comforting for me to have her support and have her hear what Dr. Ngo had to say firsthand. I was also glad that my mom and Randy were coming, too. The more support I had, the better I felt. Randy was to leave work early and meet us at Dr. Ngo's office, while Kathryn, my mom, and I drove together.

The three of us were seated in the waiting room shortly before Randy arrived. I couldn't help but notice the four hard covered books he had in his hands when he walked in the door. "What are these?" I asked pointing to the books.

"Books on radiation. I went to the library during my lunch hour and did some research. I picked up a few books so we could educate ourselves on the treatment," he said.

"I can't believe you did that. That's so sweet," I said giving him a quick peck on the lips.

Randy and I paged through the books until my name was called. The four of us stood up in unison and were led into a rather large room with enough chairs to accommodate all of us. We waited patiently until Dr. Ngo entered the room and introduced himself to us.

"I apologize for having so many people with me," I said, "but they're all part of my support system." I began introducing Randy, my mom, and Kathryn.

"That's great—that's great that you're all here," he said smiling. Dr. Ngo began asking me a number of personal questions: where was I born, how long had I lived in Southern California, my family history, how many children we had, etc. I answered each question as he took notes. He even asked me where I worked and what I did for a living. When I told him where I worked he asked me if I knew David Dukes, the president and COO of our company.

"Yes, of course I know David," I said, remembering that his late wife, Sammy, had a malignant brain tumor a few years earlier. I assumed that's how they may have known each other.

"By any chance, did you treat his wife Sammy?" I asked.

"Yes," he said. "She was a remarkable woman. Please make sure you give David my regards."

"I will," I said.

He went on to explain that I would be having a series of radiation treatments to the right breast. "You will have these treatments five days a week for approximately eight weeks," he said.

"Five days a week for eight weeks!" I exclaimed. "Wow, that's a lot!"

"Yes it is, but the treatment is given in short doses for a long duration.

However, there may be a point during your treatment sessions where you'll have to take a break for about a week or two in order to allow your skin to heal. How do you react to the sun? Do you burn easily?" he asked.

"I tend to burn in the first summer sun of the season. After that I'm fine and usually tan right away," I said.

"That's good. Patients with olive complexions such as yours tend to do remarkably well with the radiation. I usually prescribe Epi-foam, a topical foam-like substance that will help soothe any irritation or redness you may have," he said.

"What other side effects can I expect?"

"You may begin to feel fatigued at the mid-point of your treatment, and your breast will become slightly firmer," he said.

"Once my treatments are over, do you still think it's safe for us to have another baby?" I asked.

"You'll have to understand that the radiation is going directly to the breast, not your entire body. It would be different if you were getting radiation to your ovaries. So to answer your question, yes, it's perfectly safe, from a radiation standpoint, to have another healthy baby. However, I suggest waiting six to twelve months after you complete your treatment," he said.

Randy and I were pleased to learn that radiation therapy would not pose any risk to my becoming pregnant or to the health of our future baby.

"Our equipment is state-of-the-art and I have an excellent staff of technicians who will work with you. First we'll need to get a set of CT chest x-rays so we can accurately map out the precise location to radiate. To ensure the exact location is radiated each time, we tattoo dot markers the size of a pencil tip onto your breast. They're so small, only you'll be able to notice them," he said.

"We have plans to go back to Wisconsin for Christmas. Can we still go?" I asked.

"I certainly wouldn't want to spoil your fun. We can begin treatment as soon as you get back. Will you be ready to start the first week in January?" he asked.

"Yes, that would be fine," I said.

We were all impressed with Dr. Ngo's ability to put us at ease—he was so personable, warm, and friendly. After my consultation with him, I had no fears about undergoing treatment.

As we were leaving, Kathryn made a good point. She said, "Nancy, David wouldn't have sent his wife to just anyone. I'm sure he did a lot of research to find the best care for Sammy. I think you're in really good hands."

"I couldn't agree more!"

The very next morning I called David at work and reached his voice mail. I left him a message telling him about my recent diagnosis with breast cancer and how I was referred to see Dr. Ngo, who sent his regards.

When David called me back he was very sympathetic. I knew he was a compassionate man as he was very active in the "Make A Wish Foundation," which grants young children with cancer an opportunity to fulfill their wishes. After losing his wife to cancer, he was well aware of the trauma I had been going through.

"You hang in there Sunshine," he said. "You're in very good hands. I checked out several facilities all over the country and little did I know that one of the best was right here in our own backyard. If there's anything—anything at all that I can do to help you out, please let me know," he said.

He even went as far as asking me the names of all my doctors to ensure that I had the best medical care professionals. I was deeply touched that a man of his caliber would take the time out of his busy schedule to reach out and extend a helping hand to me.

My mom's visit was now coming to an end. She was ready to fly back to Wisconsin to prepare for our visit over the Christmas holiday. I was so looking forward to our vacation and could hardly wait to see all of my relatives and friends. Besides, many of them had never met our son David—including my grandma Arshelious, my dad's mother.

The following week I attended a support group for women under the age of 40 with breast cancer. Earlene, the nurse from Dr. Baick's office, told me about the group after my lumpectomy. She said it's one of the few groups in the area designed specifically for young women. I didn't feel like I really needed the support, but did feel unique since I was so young to have this cancer. I wanted an opportunity to meet other young women who had breast cancer so I wouldn't feel so alone and singled out.

When I arrived at the meeting, I was surprised to see about a dozen young women all sitting in chairs that formed into a circle. I sat down across from the facilitator. As I waited for the meeting to start, I glanced around at the other young women who were also seated, thinking how one would never know they all had cancer.

When the meeting began, the facilitator introduced herself to the group for those of us who were new. She had each of us take turns telling everyone in the group who we were, what our circumstances were, and what we hoped to achieve from the meeting.

Everyone had a story, and at the age of 35, I certainly wasn't one of the youngest in attendance, nor the oldest. The oldest woman had just turned 40. She was an attractive woman with two children, ages four and six. She shared her circumstances with the group and I was surprised to hear that she had just had a *double* mastectomy and was in the process of having reconstructive surgery. I thought she was so brave.

Another woman was 37 years old, also with two young children. She was diagnosed with invasive breast cancer one year prior, and had a lumpectomy followed by chemotherapy and radiation. She appeared to be a regular in the group, and one of the more positive ones. She spoke in an upbeat and positive manner to those in the group who were having difficulty coping. She made light of her chemotherapy experience and told us funny stories about her hair loss experience that made everyone in the group laugh.

One woman told us how upset she became after reading an article about breast cancer and learning that the percentage of survival was lower than what she had thought. Another woman quickly came to her defense and advised all of us not to get caught up in statistics or percentages of survival and reoccurrence rates from doctors or articles that we may read. "Those are just numbers—they don't mean you," she said. She had a good point. I know that if I didn't have favorable numbers, I'd get caught up in them too—I think it's only natural. However, even if the percentages of reoccurrence are low, there's still no guarantee. That's the terrible thing about this disease.

About 20 minutes into the meeting, another young woman named Liz arrived late into our session sobbing with a box of tissues in her hand. She was tall, slender and very attractive. "I apologize for being late," she said sniffling, "I've had an awful day." The facilitator asked her if she'd like to talk about it now, because she was obviously hurting. "I'm not ready to talk yet. I need some more time to calm down," said Liz.

A few more women shared their stories and then it was my turn. "My name is Nancy Madey. This is my first time here. I was diagnosed with breast cancer shortly before Thanksgiving. It came as an enormous shock because there is no history of breast cancer in my family. The worst part of it all is that I have a five-month-old baby. Fortunately, my cancer is non-invasive. I had a lumpectomy and axillary node dissection; 17 lymph nodes removed, and they were all cancer-free."

Just as I finished my sentence, Liz began wailing. The woman sitting next to Liz tried to console her. "I'll be okay," she said grabbing a tissue out of her box. "Just give me a few more minutes." The facilitator asked me to continue so I went on to say that I was going to begin radiation treatments the first week in January.

Liz was finally ready to speak. The room was quiet as we all waited to hear what was troubling her. She said she was a 28-year-old mother with a two-year-old daughter and a three-year-old son. Her cancer was not detected until the latest stage—Stage 4. By then her cancer was full-blown. She'd had a mastectomy and 12 of her 25 lymph nodes that were removed contained cancer cells.

It was now clear to all of us why her day had been awful, and why she burst into tears when I said that all 17 of my lymph nodes were cancer-free. I felt just terrible—I wanted to cry with her.

She said that she had undergone several doses of chemotherapy, and the doctors were having difficulty getting her into remission. She said she was sick of fighting and sick of wearing a wig. She just wanted her life back.

She mentioned that she was going to begin a new program the next week offered through the City of Hope in Pasadena, California, that involved stem-cell transplants, which is similar to a bone marrow transplant.

I know there wasn't a person in the room whose heart didn't go out to her. At that moment we all realized that our problems were small in comparison. Liz was literally fighting for her life and she had two young children who needed her. We all did our best to give her the support and encouragement she so desperately needed. None of us wanted her to give up fighting.

When the session was over, her husband and two young children came in to the meeting room to pick her up. I felt even worse after having seen them all—they were such a beautiful family.

After the meeting, I was emotionally distressed. I collapsed on the couch as soon as I entered our front door.

"Nancy, what's wrong?" asked Randy. "Are you okay?"

"No, I'm not okay. I just came back from a support group meeting for young women with breast cancer. I feel worse now than I did before I left. Everyone's situation was far worse than mine. It made me feel terrible—like I had no business even being there."

"What happened?" he asked. I went on to explain what had occurred at the meeting.

"Maybe this isn't for you Nancy," he said. "It seems to me like it's making you feel depressed and causing you to think about this problem more than you should."

"I think you're right. I'm emotionally exhausted."

"Support groups are great for a lot of people but they're not for everyone. Some people are alone or don't have the love and support from family and friends like you do. It's mainly designed for people like that, or for people with cancer who really want to help others. Give it a rest Nancy."

Randy was right. From that day on I chose not to attend another breast cancer support group. I thought that was the best thing I could have done for *me* at the time.

* * * * * * * * * *

Christmas was approaching quickly. I was excited to go to Wisconsin and spend the holiday with my family and friends. It's what I really needed—a chance to get away and experience a different change of pace. Since this was going to be little David's first time on an airplane, we chose to take a direct flight from Orange County to Chicago. Once in Chicago, we rented a car and drove to Racine, Wisconsin, as opposed to taking a small puddle jumper from Chicago to Milwaukee and then driving to Racine.

David was extremely good on the plane—he never fussed. Those who were seated around us commented on how good he was.

"Is he always that good?" a middle-age woman asked.

"Well, actually he is. We've been blessed with a little angel," I said.

When the plane landed we got our luggage and picked up our rental car. The drive from Chicago to Racine was about 90 minutes. Fortunately, there wasn't any snow to cause hazardous driving conditions.

When we drove up the driveway of my mother's house she came run ning outside to greet us. She took David into the house right away so as not expose him to the bitter cold any longer than necessary, while Randy and I brought in the luggage.

This was going to be my first Christmas at my parent's house since my dad passed away—so, naturally it was going to feel different. David's presence helped to fill the void we all felt by bringing a smile to everyone's face—babies have a way of doing that. This was David's first Christmas— the Christmas when he would meet his only surviving great grandparent for the first time, my grandma Arshelious.

On Christmas Eve we attended an evening worship at church with Father Yeprem officiating. He talked openly and freely with the congregation, asking us to recall and give thanks to God for those things with which we have all been blessed. He asked if any of us would like to share our thanks aloud. I felt moved—like I needed to proclaim my experience and glorify God for helping me through a very trying time. I was the first to speak aloud. "I'm thankful for our beautiful son, and for God's help in getting me through my recent diagnosis of breast cancer."

Many of the parish members were surprised to hear my message of thanks, and came up to me after the service saying they would pray for me. Father Yeprem gave me a big hug and said he was happy to see I was doing so well, and would continue to pray for me.

The following day was Christmas. Family, relatives, and friends filled my mother's house as she hosted a wonderful Christmas dinner with a variety of special dishes and desserts. My brother Tod was there too; however, my sister Kathy and her husband Jeff, from Colorado, were spending the holiday in Florida with Jeff's family. My aunts, uncles, cousins and Grandma came to share the Christmas joy.

The highlight of my Christmas was seeing my grandma hold David in her arms. I could tell how proud she was to witness this new generation of life—a generation which she had hoped her own son (my dad) could have seen.

Grandma never knew about *my* cancer. I felt that it was something she could do without knowing. She had been through enough in the past two years with her son's illness and ultimate demise. Grandma also lost her husband to whom she was married for 71 years, just four months prior to losing her first-born son.

Those at our family gathering commented on how different our Christmases were without my dad, for he was the liveliest one in the family. He'd spend time playing with the kids and joking around with the adults—his presence was definitely missed.

Every Christmas Eve for as long as I can remember, we'd have a huge family celebration at my grandpa and grandma Mikaelian's house, in conjunction with their wedding anniversary, which actually was on Christmas Eve.

We'd been celebrating together for over two decades. Uncle Sam would organize an open house—an opportunity for friends and family members to gather and celebrate Christmas as well as my grandparents' wedding anniversary. We'd have hors d'oeuvres, and a variety of entrees, desserts and beverages. Some of my best family memories are from Christmases at Grandpa and Grandma's house.

Then, after our Christmas dinner, Uncle Sam would haul a huge box of gifts into the living room and distribute beautifully wrapped packages to all of his nieces and nephews. This annual tradition was kept alive until shortly before my grandpa passed away in 1993. I often wish that I could go back and relive those moments—only this time with Randy and David.

I also got to see a few of my cousin's children for the first time. They were all close to David in age. It was a joy having a house full of babies at Christmas time.

Our vacation went by so quickly, and before we knew it, it was time to head back to California. I was somewhat anxious to go back and begin my radiation treatments so I could move on with my life. I just wanted it all to be over.

6

After the New Year, I had an appointment with one of Dr. Ngo's technicians. His name was Bill, and he was responsible for mapping out the exact areas of my breast that were to be treated. In doing so, he had me lie down on a simulation table (similar to the table used during radiation) to plot out the area of my breast that required radiation. I could see all of my x-rays hanging up on the viewing box. He told me that if I were to receive the same amount of radiation to my entire body, as I would be getting to my breast, it would literally kill me. Since it's concentrated to the breast area only, it wouldn't. That was one piece of information I could have done without. However, it made me realize just how powerful radiation truly is.

The mapping procedure was very scientific, requiring a computer and a lot of high-tech equipment. He began mapping out the locations on my breast with a red and black magic marker. He'd draw different sizes of circles and X's over all over my right breast. By the time he was done, my breast looked like an abstract piece of art. I laughed and told him that he ought to sign his name to his masterpiece.

When he was finished, Dr. Ngo came in and reviewed the films and his work.

"Okay, it looks like we'll give you your tattoos tomorrow and we can start your radiation treatments on Monday," Dr. Ngo said.

After I got dressed, Bill told me not to wash off the ink marks he had drawn on my breast and to let them wear off naturally. Then he scheduled me for a series of radiation appointments, Monday through Friday at 8:30 a.m. He said the radiation treatment time would be less than a minute, but I would need about ten to 15 minutes total time in which to undress, get positioned, marked and radiated.

The next day I went in to get tattooed. It was fast, simple, and painless. Just a quick pin prick with a needle in six locations and it was done! Now, whenever I have conversations with others about tattoos, I can say I have SIX and leave the rest up to their imaginations!

I called Marcia to tell her that my medical leave would soon be over and I'd be returning to the office next week. She was thrilled. I told her that I'd be having radiation treatments on a set schedule—8:30 a.m. for the next eight weeks. "We're all anxious to have you back," she said. "I'll see you on Monday."

Monday morning I arrived at West Coast Radiology Center, ready to begin my first radiation treatment. I signed in at the receptionist's desk and waited to be called. There were a few other people in the waiting room, and I knew they could only be there for one reason—radiation treatments.

When my name was called, I was told to take the elevator down the hall to the lower basement level. How eerie, I thought—the basement. The elevators opened in the lower level and a technician who was about my age greeted me.

"Hi, my name is Ramin, and I'll be your technician for the next eight weeks along with Annemarie. Annemarie—where are you?" he asked.

"Here I am," she said. "I'm the one who pushes the buttons behind the wall, and Ramin is the one who positions you on the table to align you with the radiation beam," she said.

Why couldn't it be the other way around, I thought. I felt uncomfortable about having to bare my breast to a guy who was probably younger than I! Oh well, I gotta do what I gotta do, I told myself.

"Let me take you back, show you the equipment and explain what we'll be doing to you over the next several weeks," Ramin said, walking toward a solid cement wall.

Behind the wall was an enormous, dimly lit room without any windows. There were several huge pieces of equipment that I had never seen before. And why would I have? I never had radiation before. Ramin explained that I'd have to lie down on what looked like an examination table. He showed me how he could raise the table up, down, and sideways to accurately position me according to the locations of my tattoos.

"Do you treat a lot of breast cancer patients?" I asked.

"We treat all kinds of cancer patients, and have had way too many breast cancer patients," he said.

"Are they as young as I?" I asked, wondering if I was the only young woman who would be exposing her breasts to him.

"Some are even younger than you," he said. "After I position you on the table, I'll turn the lights off and leave the room. You'll need to stay perfectly still and try not to move. There's a gown in the dressing room. Remove everything from the waist up and when you're ready just come right out."

"Okay," I said as I walked toward the dressing rooms. I undressed from the waist up just as he had said, put on the hospital gown, and walked out of the dressing room back to where the radiation equipment was. To my surprise Dr. Ngo was there, too.

"Hi Nancy. It's good to see you again. I won't be here every time you have your treatment, but it's my standard practice to come down on my patient's first day," he said. "Every Wednesday after your radiation treatment, you'll come back upstairs so I can examine you. I want to see how your skin is reacting to the treatment, as well as get a blood sample from you so we can monitor your white blood cell count and your platelets."

"I'm fine with that," I said, as Ramin began positioning me on the table. I tried not to be embarrassed and kept telling myself that he's in the medical profession and this is his job. I figured I'd have to get over the embarrassment quickly if I was going to see him five days a week for eight weeks.

"Now lie still and don't move," he said as he turned the lights off and left the room.

I heard a faint sizzling sound. That must be the radiation I thought. Before I knew it, he turned the lights on and was back in the room.

"You can get dressed now," he said helping me down off the table. "That's it?"

"That's it," he said.

"Okay, I'll see you tomorrow." I said good bye to Annemarie, and headed back to the dressing room to change back into my suit. I was excited to go back to work, as I had been off for six weeks. I was beginning to get a little bored at home and wanted to fill my thoughts with things other than cancer.

My office was only a five-minute drive from the radiation center, which made for an easy commute. I started to feel strange as I pulled into the parking lot. I began to wonder if word had gotten around that I had breast cancer. I'm sure all of my associates wondered where I was and why I had been out of the office for so long. I made no stipulations to Marcia or my friends at work about keeping my illness private. My life was an open book (pun intended!). In fact, I *wanted* people to know, especially the women. I wanted them to be aware of this disease, to do their monthly breast exams and have their annual mammograms. I wanted them to know that I had no family history of breast cancer, and that this could happen to them as easily as it happened to me. I just wanted to educate them.

When I got to the office, it was decorated with balloons and a "Welcome Back" sign. My assistants came running up to me, telling me how glad they were to have me back. In no time at all, everyone was standing outside my cubicle welcoming me back and asking how I was doing. The warm greetings made me feel really special.

Before I knew it, it was back to business as usual. I had a lot of paperwork to review and phone calls to return. Marcia caught me up on the status of my projects, and assigned me a few more.

Throughout the day, associates from various departments would pass me in the hall—I couldn't help but wonder if they knew. They had to have heard, I thought to myself. News like that spreads like wildfire.

Others who had heard that I had been diagnosed with breast cancer stopped by my office to ask how I was doing and welcome me back. Lots of people kept telling me how good I looked. I didn't mind, but I'm sure I couldn't have changed that much in six weeks! Did they expect me to look different? I think they just didn't know what to say, and wanted to say something nice to make me feel good.

Even Janet, the vice president of our department, stopped by my office and gave me a warm welcome back hug. That meant a lot to me. She genuinely cared. She had even called me at home a few times, which really touched me. She told me that her mother-in-law had breast cancer that was treated by radiation, and was doing fine.

I found that those people who had family members or loved ones stricken with this disease were far more compassionate. Many people would share cancer survival stories about their mothers, fathers, grandparents, aunts, uncles, sisters, brothers, husbands, wives, and even themselves.

The more I opened up to people at work about my own experience with breast cancer, the more they confided in me about their own personal battles with other types of cancer. Some of the people with such experiences were even younger than I!

Having become so aware of the risks of this disease, I started performing self-breast exams just as Dr. Mahmood had instructed me to do. I remembered him saying to check as high up as my collarbone—which I did. One time my hand went a little further and I found a lump along the base of my neck. I immediately thought that I had another occurrence of cancer, and perhaps it was lymphoma like my dad had. "Please God," I said aloud, "Don't let it be more cancer!"

I showed Randy what I had discovered, and he suggested that I have Dr. Ngo look at it the next day when I went for my weekly exam. I was hopeful that I would be able to get this resolved once and for all. I couldn't go on the rest of my life living in fear, thinking that every lump I found in my body was going to be cancerous.

After the radiation treatment on Wednesday, I went to see Dr. Ngo for my weekly exam. He said I was doing fine. I pointed out the lump I had found on my neck and asked him to take a look at it. He began feeling both sides of my neck and didn't say anything. The longer he examined me the more fearful I became.

"Dr. Ngo, is this something I should be worried about?" I asked, hoping he'd say no.

"We worry about all of our patients. Let's wait a few more weeks and keep an eye on it," he said. It could just be a normal lymph node. Have you been sick with a cold recently?"

"Yes, but that was weeks ago. Now I'm doubly scared. My dad died of lymphoma. I can't wait a few weeks Dr. Ngo, I have to know NOW," I said crying. "I can't go through this again. Can't you do an ultrasound or something?" I asked in desperation.

He could see how distraught I was and offered to order a MRI (Magnetic Resonance Imaging). A MRI is a painless procedure like an x-ray, which involves the use of a powerful magnet to transmit radio waves through the body. The images appear on a computer screen as well as on film. This procedure would determine exactly what was in my neck.

I was scheduled to go back the next day for the test. He told me he'd call me the following day with the results.

After that appointment, I went back to work and immediately went to Laura's desk and told her about the new lump I found and the MRI appointment.

"Nancy, that's almost impossible! What are the odds that you'd get breast cancer, and then develop lymphoma within two months of each other?" she asked. Laura always had a way of putting things into perceptive to calm my nerves. "You're going to be fine."

I went back to my desk and called Randy at work. I told him about my conversation with Dr. Ngo and that I was going to have an MRI.

"I'm sure it's nothing, Nancy," he said, trying to console me.

"As far as I'm concerned, there is no such thing as *nothing* anymore. My last *nothing* turned out to be breast cancer! I think that's *something*!"

I was all choked up and could barely speak. "I gotta go," I said as I hung up the phone.

That evening Randy could tell I was upset. "I'm going to take the afternoon off and be with you," he said.

"That's not necessary. Maybe you can just come home after the procedure instead," I said. "Waiting at home alone for Dr. Ngo's phone call will be agonizing."

I could barely sleep that night. I felt like my formerly normal life was just snowballing into one of complete chaos. I worked through my lunch hour the next day and then left the office at 1:15 p.m. for the radiology center. Once I arrived, I signed in and waited about ten minutes before I was called.

"Here's a gown," said one of the technicians. "Undress from head to toe, except for your panties. When you're ready, just walk right through those double doors," she said, pointing to a set of white doors. When I went through the doors, she told me to lie down on the exam table.

"We're going to inject a dye into your system so that the area will show up on the MRI. Are you claustrophobic?" she asked.

"No."

"Good, then you shouldn't have a problem once you're inside the cylinder," she said. She started getting ready to inject my right arm when I quickly pulled away, remembering that I had to protect that arm.

"I had an axillary node dissection," I said, "so you'll have to inject the dye in my left arm. I was recently diagnosed with breast cancer and had to get some lymph nodes removed."

"Were any of your lymph nodes involved?" she asked.

"No, thank God. I had 17 removed and they were all negative."

She shook her head and said, "More and more young women are getting diagnosed with breast cancer every day. It's pretty scary."

"Tell me about it."

"I need you to relax now while I inject the dye into your arm. You may feel a warm tingly sensation as it goes in. That's perfectly normal."

Once she finished administering the dye into my arm, she asked me to lie on another table, which would then be entered into a tunnel-like cylinder. I did as she asked and was finished in less than ten minutes.

I put my clothes on and went straight home. My head was is another world. I hated taking tests where I had to wait for results. I'd done that too many times in the past few months. I couldn't bear the thought of doing it again, but I had no choice.

Randy came home from work about an hour after I arrived. He walked in the door with a beautiful bouquet of fresh flowers for me.

"I thought you might like these," he said.

"Randy, they're beautiful. You didn't have to do that."

I put the flowers in a vase and asked what he wanted to do for dinner.

"Let's just order a pizza or something. Does that sound good to you?"

"Well, I'm really not that hungry. I feel like I can't function until I have the results. Feel my hands," I said putting them out for him to touch. "Do you feel how clammy they are? I'm so nervous."

Since David was napping, we worked on a puzzle to pass the time. It was nearly 5 p.m. and I still hadn't received a call from Dr. Ngo.

"Why don't you just call Dr. Ngo's office before they close and find out if the results are in?" Randy suggested.

I picked up the phone and called his office. I told the receptionist who I was and asked if I could speak to Dr. Ngo. When Dr. Ngo came on the phone, he told me that he was still waiting for the results and should have them within the next 30 minutes. "I know how anxious you must feel," he said.

About 20 minutes later, the phone rang. My heart began to race even more. This phone call was going to determine my destiny.

"Hello."

"Nancy, it's Dr. Ngo. You're fine. The test showed that it was just a normal lymph node. I'll see you next week. Enjoy the rest of your evening."

"Oh, I will," I said hanging up the phone. I literally began jumping up and down in the living room shouting, "I'm okay! I'm okay! I'm okay!"

"I knew you would be Nancy," Randy said giving me a big hug and kiss.

"I felt like I could have died twice within a few months. First with the breast cancer, and then this."

"Yeah, and you're scaring me to death in the process. Nancy, you're going to out-live us all." Just then, David awoke from his nap. I think he must have heard me jumping up and down in ecstasy. I ran upstairs to get him. He was so happy to see me. I picked him up out of the crib and cradled him in my arms. "Mama loves you and will never leave you," I whispered in his tiny ears. That night *I* slept like a baby! I continued with the radiation treatments. By the sixth week I was beginning to feel fatigued. The demands of my job and my baby were more than I could handle. I could no longer do what I was accustomed to doing and often cried out of despair. I felt overwhelmed and out of control.

Dr. Ngo suggested that I take a break from radiation for a few weeks because my skin was getting very irritated. He gave me a prescription for Epi-foam, which would help soothe the burning sensation I was experiencing on my breast. He recommended that I didn't wear a bra and take another medical leave (which I did) until I felt strong enough to go back to work.

During the medical leave, I relaxed and read a few health books. Having had breast cancer made me realize that I should make some dramatic lifestyle changes—changes to help me become healthier and live longer. I've always been on the slender side and had difficulty putting on weight. I knew that I needed to incorporate more fruits and vegetables into my diet and eat less meat. One book I read suggested using vegetables as a main entree, and meat as a garnish. Another book I read explained the different types vitamins and minerals that helped to reduce the risk of cancer. I started applying what I learned, but never got to the point of obsession.

I also knew I needed to work on my mental health. I needed to learn how to be calm and not "sweat the small stuff." After reading several books on the topic, I put a list of bullet points on a small card to pull out and refer to whenever I found myself feeling stressed or worried. Here's how the list read:

How can I *under-react* to downplay this situation? Tell myself:
- This is no big deal
- This will pass
- It's just anxiety
- It will go away
- This is not worth getting upset over
- Don't sweat the small stuff

- One year from now this won't matter
- One year from now I won't remember this
- It's not the end of the world
- It just doesn't matter
- This is not an emergency
- It's not my problem
- It's only money
- So what!

I shared the list with several of my friends, all of whom liked it and asked for a copy. I still have the list posted on our refrigerator at home.

Another way I tried to reduce stress was through yoga. I took a class and found it to be very relaxing. It helped me to get in touch with my inner soul by generating a calmness and feeling of inner peace.

By the end of February, I began to notice that my energy level was slowly returning. The radiation treatments were finally over! The radiation center gave me a red rose and a diploma stating that I had graduated from radiation therapy. I truly felt like I had reached a major milestone in my life.

7

It was finally over! I went to battle and won the war. Now it was time to shift gears and map out a new lifestyle, one filled with balance and harmony. That was critical. Something had to change and I owed it to myself and my family to make that change. Failure to do so would cause me to revert back to an old, unhealthy pattern of stress brought on by overachieving. I couldn't allow myself to do that—especially after everything I had just been through.

A part-time job was the answer to providing the balance and harmony that I craved. Upon returning to work in May after my medical leave, I had a clear vision of what I wanted and what I needed to accomplish. I was determined to make it work—even if it meant leaving the company and foregoing a promotion I had been promised. I was very open and honest with my boss Marcia, and immediately discussed my desire to work part-time. She was empathetic to the change I wanted to make; unfortunately, it could not be done. Marcia believed that the demands of the job and the amount of responsibility it entailed was full-time.

Marcia offered to help me obtain my goal, and gave me suggestions as to how I should peruse a part-time job or a job-share opportunity within the company. "The company is growing rapidly," she said. "Soon there's going to be a need to create new positions—perhaps even parttime. I'll keep my eyes and ears open for you," she said.

"Thanks Marcia. I'd really appreciate that."

In less than two weeks, Marcia told me that our company had just acquired a division of another organization just outside of Denver. She said positions were to be opening up at our facility to help transition and grow this new division. Marcia said she had already spoken to Rick, the senior director and general manager of the newly created department, and he seemed interested in me.

"I told Rick that I'd have you call him," she said with a smile on her face.

"Really? I can't believe how fast this is happening! Thanks Marcia."

When I called Rick, he briefly explained the position to me. "It will involve generating marketing plans and business presentations, as well as being responsible for our reseller database," he said.

"Well, it certainly sounds like something I would enjoy doing and be good at," I said.

We set up an appointment for the interview, and he asked me to bring a copy of my resume, as well as some of my writing samples, to our meeting. I was so excited! I couldn't believe how nicely everything was falling into place. I felt confident of my abilities, and was eager to learn more about the position.

A week later I had the interview with Rick. It went extremely well. He asked me what my reasons were for wanting to pursue a part-time position. I was very honest and direct as to why I wanted to make a change.

"I was recently diagnosed with breast cancer," I said. "Although I'm now cancer-free, I decided to make some lifestyle changes and choosing to work part-time is one of the changes." Rick didn't seem overly shocked when I shared my reasons with him. "In addition, I have a one-year-old son I would like to spend more time with, especially during his formative years," I said confidently.

"Well, you came highly recommended by Marcia, and I think we both could benefit if you joined our team. Let me review your writing samples and get back to you in a few days," he said. "In the meantime, you let me know what part-time days and hours will work best for you."

I was impressed with Rick's flexibility, and knew I would enjoy working with him. I also felt the experience of working on a new "start-up" operation would be invaluable.

I told Marcia the interview went well and it sounded as if the job were tailor-made for me. "Rick would be lucky to have you," she said.

Within a few weeks, Rick called and offered me the position. I was thrilled! Human Resources will be contacting you to present your offer letter. Should you choose to accept the offer, I'd like you to start July 15th," he said.

"That would be fine," I said excitedly.

"Have you decided what days and hours you'd like to work?" he asked.

"Yes. I'd like to work Tuesdays, Wednesdays, and Thursdays; eight hours a day."

"Oh, so you'll have a four-day weekend every week. Won't that be nice?" he said with a chuckle.

For once in my life, I felt like I was privileged. Having the opportunity to work part-time in a managerial capacity was almost unheard of, yet the company was willing to make it work for me. Soon I would have the best of both worlds—an opportunity to remain in the work force and spend more time with David. I was now on my way to obtaining the balance and harmony I so badly wanted.

I continued getting blood tests every three months as part of the follow-up program with Dr. Baick. In addition to the blood tests, he recommended that I have a mammogram in June (which was six months after my initial diagnosis), and then every year thereafter.

It was now June, 1997, and I was ready to have my first mammogram after completing my initial treatment. I was somewhat nervous, but was told that West Coast Radiology Center is sensitive to the emotions of cancer patients. They actually provide each patient with her results before she leaves the center. I was thankful for that.

The mammogram was more painful this time, but only on the radiated breast. This was because my breast had become firm and less pliable after the radiation, just as Dr. Ngo had predicted.

Before I could put my clothes back on and begin to wonder what the outcome would be, the technician came in the examination room and told me that everything was fine! An instant sigh of relief came over me. Thank God!

Randy and all of my family members and friends were overjoyed about my clean bill of health. It was a very happy time for all of us.

On June 7 we celebrated David's first birthday. He was just starting to walk and was taking a few steps by himself. I was elated to be healthy and thrilled to be a part of all of his milestones.

Once I started my part-time job, I knew I had made the right decision. I appreciated having Mondays and Fridays off and enjoyed spending those days with David. I tried hard to make up for the time I had lost with him during my bout with cancer—the times when I couldn't lift him up and hold him in my arms, the times when I was physically too tired to play with him, and the times I couldn't share fun activities with him. Although I knew I could never get those moments back, I made every effort to try. I'd lift him, hold him, and play with him. I'd smother him with hugs and kisses every chance I had.

We'd do fun things like go to the beach, the zoo, and the park. We'd spend countless hours playing on the swings, the teeter-totter, and the slide. I'd take him on long walks in his stroller and point out objects along the way for him to learn. I spent time teaching him the names of animals, colors, and how to count. I'd read to him, sing to him, and play with him as much as I possibly could. It was good for both of us. We were enjoying the time together—the time that we would not have had, had I still been working 40 hours a week.

As a family, we started traveling again and took trips to Colorado, Ohio, and Wisconsin to visit our families. We vacationed in Arizona, and took weekend jaunts to Santa Barbara and San Diego. We were doing more and appreciating our time together.

That summer, my family and I were invited to an open house hosted by the hospital. The event was a tribute to all patients who survived cancer—"You're a Star" was the theme. The survivors were to bring a photograph of themselves to be placed on a huge wall. I was proud to be a survivor and I wanted to go to the event and celebrate!

Randy and I began mingling with others, eating, and enjoying the musical entertainment. In the distance I could see the wall on which all of the cancer survivors were to place photos of themselves. I excused myself from Randy, and walked over to the wall with my photograph in hand. As I looked for a place to hang the picture, I was surprised to see how many photos there were. I began looking at all of the snapshots—there were so many, mainly older individuals. Then I glanced down and saw a cluster of photos. They were pictures of children—some even younger than our son. Tears began falling down my cheeks. I was so grateful that it was I who had been diagnosed with cancer, not David. Quietly sobbing, I placed my photo on the wall, then walked away.

I was disturbed. I felt my photograph didn't belong on the wall with the rest of the cancer survivors. I felt as if I were putting myself into a category I didn't belong. Suddenly, I was reluctant to identify myself as a cancer survivor, and I didn't want my picture displayed on the wall. I walked back to the wall, and when no one was looking, I removed my photograph. I couldn't explain myself—it was just something I felt compelled to do.

I was disappointed by how emotional I had become. This was a time to be celebrating my survival, not brooding in self pity. I thought I was beyond that, but obviously I wasn't. I realized I still had some healing to do, it was just a matter of time.

That August marked the tragic death of Princess Diana. As the world reacted with sadness, shock and deep grief, so did I. Princess Diana was one of the women I had admired most. *The Death of a Princess 1961-1997*, ran across the bottom of every TV station I watched. Seeing the years 1961-1997 had a major impact on me. Princess Diana and I were born in the same year. We were the same age.

How young she was to have died, and how tragic it was for her two sons to lose their mother, I thought. I began to wonder why my life was spared, and why Princess Diana's was taken away. If anyone had a purpose in life, it was Princess Diana. The world needed her—she had such passion for people. She traveled far and wide on behalf of many causes, and was considered an international humanitarian.

What was my purpose? What was so special about my life that I had been spared by God? I pondered these questions over and over and came up with only one reason. It's part of God's master plan and I must not question His word. Although I may not know what my purpose in life is, I hope that one day I will discover it with God's help.

In the fall, Randy and I decided to seek another medical opinion about having another child—not to undermine my oncologist in anyway, but merely to get another opinion. Since there hadn't been much research done on pregnancy after breast cancer (as most women who get this disease are beyond their childbearing years), we wanted to feel comfortable knowing that my life wouldn't be in jeopardy. By starting our research early, we would know the risks involved, and could be better prepared to entertain other options, such as adoption.

My mother had suggested I contact her friend Irene, who had been diagnosed with breast cancer just six months prior to me. Several years ago she and her husband relocated from Wisconsin to California, and now she lived only a few miles from us.

"Perhaps you can get a second opinion from Irene's doctor," my mom said. "Why don't you give her a call?"

When I called Irene, she was very sad to learn of my experience, but was happy to hear I was doing well. Irene has a wonderful attitude and is very positive, despite the fact she had to undergo chemotherapy. She said she had a wonderful oncologist named Dr. Barth, who is based in Newport Beach.

I made an appointment for a consultation with Dr. Barth and submitted copies of my records and films prior to our meeting. Dr. Barth said pregnancy could pose a slight risk of developing cancer—mainly in the opposite breast. He gave us the same statistics as my oncologist Dr. Mahmood had; that if I lived to be 85 years old, I'd have a 30-percent chance of developing breast cancer or a 0.8 percent chance per year. "Choosing to have another baby is a personal decision that you and Randy are going to have to make. You'll have to decide what's comfortable for both of you," he said.

Knowing that nothing in life worth having is risk-free, we decided that we'd try to have another baby when David turned two. After all, the risk was rather low.

It's not just the individual who is affected by breast cancer, it's her family and friends too. In the United States alone, there is an estimated 178,700 new cases of breast cancer diagnosed each year, making it the second leading cause of death in women. October is "Breast Cancer Awareness" month. It is devoted to promoting awareness, remembering those who have lost their lives to breast cancer as well as those who have survived it. It's also a time for many organizations to sponsor fundraising events to raise money for research.

Sandi, my college friend who lives in Los Angeles, sent me a letter. It said, *"Last weekend I did the Revlon Breast & Ovarian Cancer 5K run.*

Here's a picture to let you know that I was thinking about you. Stay well! Stay strong! Love, Sandi." The photo she enclosed showed Sandi at the race with a pink sign on her back which said, *"I'm running in support of Nancy Madey."* I was deeply touched and started crying. I immediately picked up the phone to thank her.

My neighbor, Julie, was one in over 20,500 participants in Orange County who ran the "Race for the Cure". Her mother is a breast cancer survivor, so Julie ran the race with both of our names on her back. It's amazing how many people come together from all over the country to support such a great cause.

Although my cancer ordeal was over, the possibility of a new occurrence, or a re-occurrence, lingered in the back of my mind. I was never truly at peace. I always had an underlying fear that I might have to face a similar experience in the future. I figured if it was going to happen, it would most likely be when I was in my 50's or 60's, as that's the age it strikes most women.

In November, I celebrated the one-year anniversary of surviving cancer. I couldn't believe how quickly it came around. Randy and I went out for a nice romantic dinner—just the two of us.

After Thanksgiving, Randy suggested that the two of us sit down and write our goals for 1998. Our long-term goal was to have another child, and our short-term goal was to celebrate our four-year wedding anniversary in Maui. We also made another goal to move to Huntington Beach, our neighboring city, and buy a home. It was fun establishing our goals together—now it was just a matter of achieving them.

8

The New Year arrived—1998! Randy and I were anxious to begin achieving the goals we had set for ourselves.

Since I was responsible for managing our in-house travel department at work, I took it upon myself to plan our family vacation to Hawaii. I had taken some course work in travel at the local college, and remembered one of my classmates, Jon, was breaking into the travel industry as an agent. I thought it would be nice if I could give him our business since he was just starting out. So much had been going on in my life that I hadn't talked to him in almost a year. He was glad to hear from me and said he was enjoying his new career. I briefly told him about my breast cancer experience. He felt badly for me, but was delighted to hear that everything turned out well. I asked him if he could plan our travel for us as we wanted to spend our four-year wedding anniversary in Maui (with David). I provided him with the dates and he said he'd get right on it.

By March, our real estate agent had found us a beautiful four-bedroom, two-story home just a few miles from the ocean in Huntington Beach. It was spacious and definitely a home we could grow into. Randy and I really liked it, and told our real estate agent that we'd like to make an offer. My mom and my sister Kathy, who were both out visiting, thought the home was beautiful too. We were hopeful that our goal of buying a home would soon be within reach.

Although my next mammogram wasn't actually due until June, I decided to push it up a few months and schedule it the end of March, in conjunction with my three-month check-up with Dr. Baick. My mom offered to watch David and I asked Kathy to accompany me to the appointment for moral support.

I was glad Kathy came with me, as she helped to alleviate the little nervousness I had. When I was called, I went in while my sister sat in the waiting room. The technician handed me a hospital gown and told me to undress from the waist up. When I was ready, she escorted me into the room for the mammogram.

First the technician positioned my radiated breast on the cold metal plate, as another cold metal plate came clamping down. She asked me to take a deep breath and then repeated the procedure on my left side. I remembered the center's policy to inform cancer patients of their results prior to them leaving, so I didn't feel terribly over-anxious. Besides, my oncologist Dr. Mahmood had said the odds of getting a new occurrence of breast cancer was only 0.8 percent per year. Since this was my first year, the odds of developing cancer again would be extremely low.

The technician took the films and told me to wait a few minutes until the radiologist reviewed them. When the technician came back she said that she needed to redo the left side. I was beginning to feel somewhat paranoid.

"Redo the left side?" My heart began to skip a beat. "Why?" I asked. "We didn't get a good picture," she said as she continued adjusting my breast. "Now take a deep breath and hold. OK, you can release now. I'll be right back," she said as she left the room.

I waited, with sweaty palms, until the technician returned. "You can see Dr. Baick for your next appointment now," she said.

"Is everything alright?" I asked.

"Dr. Baick will go over everything with you," she said taking me to one of the examination rooms. "I understand you brought your sister with you. Would you like me to get her from the waiting room and have her here with you?" she asked.

"Sure," I said, wondering if the technician knew something and was keeping it from me.

"I'll be right back."

I was very happy to see Kathy come into the examination room. I briefly told her what I had just experienced. Before she could respond, Dr. Baick entered the room with my file in his hands and introduced himself to Kathy.

"I just finished reviewing your films and noticed that you have micro-calcifications on your left breast. Calcifications that didn't appear on your last mammogram a year ago," Dr. Baick said.

My heart sunk down to my stomach. I began to panic and shake. Kathy moved closer and gently put her arm around me. "What does that mean?" I asked with deep concern.

"Well, it could be that they are just normal calcifications. However, they weren't present on your last mammogram. Since you're considered a high-risk patient, it's my job to determine exactly what it is," he said. "We'll have to surgically remove the tissue and get a biopsy."

I started bawling. "I can't go through this again, Dr. Baick. I've been through so much!" I exclaimed. "Plus we're in the process of buying a house...what am I suppose to do?"

"Don't do anything different. There's only a 20-percent chance it's cancer, but I have to be sure. Come with me," he said.

Kathy and I followed him to another room where my films were hanging up on a view box.

"This is your mammogram from last year, and this is your mammogram from today," he said pointing to several tiny white dots. "These are what we believe to be microscopic calcifications. As you can see, they didn't appear on your mammogram from last June," he said.

"Where will the incision be?" I asked quivering.

"It will be a horizontal incision from the outer side, approximately one to one-and-a-half inches toward the center."

My hands and knees were shaking badly. Dr. Baick and Kathy noticed how I was trembling, and they both wrapped their arms around me and gave me a hug.

"Please don't worry until we know for sure. We see these types of things often and they're usually normal," he said as we slowly walked back into the examination room.

Just hearing the word "biopsy" made me cringe. It meant waiting another four days for the pathology report. Another four days of Hell.

"Earlene will arrange a date and time for your surgery. She'll be in shortly to explain the procedure to you," he said.

My sister put her arm around my shoulder, assuring me that everything would be all right.

"I've had calcifications show up on my mammograms too. It's nothing to worry about," she said, trying her best to console me.

"Promise me you won't tell Mom," I said. "I've already put her through enough."

"Okay, but I think you'll feel better if you tell her. She can handle it—there is an 80-percent chance that it's *not* cancer," Kathy said.

"I still don't want her to know. Please promise me."

"I promise," she said reluctantly.

Earlene tapped on the door as she walked in. "I have your surgery scheduled for Tuesday. That's tomorrow, March 31st at 7:30 a.m. You'll need to arrive at the hospital by 6 in the morning for prep work. Does that work for you?"

"Yes, I'll make it work," I said.

"Here's a list of instructions for you to follow," she said handing me a piece of paper. "Make sure you begin fasting at midnight the night before, and don't have anything to eat or drink the next morning. As far as the procedure is concerned, since the area in question is microscopic, they'll have to do a needle localization mammogram. A needle will be inserted into the side of your left breast, and will remain in your breast during surgery. The needle will serve as a guide for Dr. Baick to locate and remove the microscopic tissue."

At this point I wasn't sure what I heard and didn't really care. All I could think about was having to experience another episode of waiting for biopsy results. This just didn't seem fair! I had already gone through enough for someone my age. I just wanted the chaos to end!

After I got dressed, I asked Earlene if I could use one of their private offices to call my husband at work and tell him. She took Kathy and me to a nearby office and told me to take my time.

Luckily, Randy was in his office when I called. He knew I was going in for my mammogram and three-month follow-up that day, but hadn't thought it was anything for us to be concerned about.

"Randy, it's me. I'm calling from Dr. Baick's office. I had a bad mammogram."

I heard nothing but silence on the other end. "Randy, are you there?" I asked.

"Yeah, I'm here," he said silently listening for what I was about to say next.

"Dr. Baick found some calcifications that …," I got choked up and couldn't speak. I began to cry and handed the phone to Kathy.

Kathy explained to Randy that Dr. Baick said there was only a 20-percent chance that it was cancer, and not to worry. She went on to tell him that I needed to have another biopsy and the surgery was scheduled for tomorrow morning. When she noticed I had calmed down, she handed the phone back to me.

"I want to talk to Dr. Baick," Randy demanded.

"Randy, there's nothing to discuss!" I exclaimed. "This is very stressful for me—can we talk about it when you come home tonight?"

"Of course we can, but I'd like more details from Dr. Baick," he said.

"I'm telling you everything I know," I said sniffling. "I'm sorry to be dumping this on you while you're at work, but I needed to hear your voice."

"We'll get through it, Love, don't worry."

After I hung up the phone with Randy, I called my boss, Rick, to let him know that I wouldn't be in the office tomorrow or the remainder of the workweek. Unfortunately I got his voice mail, but I left him a detailed message. I told him I'd call him after I had the results of the biopsy, and asked him to pray for me.

I gathered my things, and before I left, Margo, one of Dr. Baick's medical assistants, gave me a hug. "Please don't worry," she said. In spite of everything, her hug was very consoling.

I hardly spoke to my sister the entire car ride home. I was numb. I was afraid. I needed time to process what had just happened. I can't go through this again, I thought. But I knew I had to come to terms with it, because I did indeed have to go through it again. I needed to hope for the best and prepare for the worst—all over again, and all too soon. My mental and emotional stamina was destroyed. I didn't think I could face Round 2!

When we got home, I went to the refrigerator and poured a glass of soda. David was playing with some blocks on the floor. I got down on my knees and helped him stack the blocks. He giggled as he deliberately knocked them over.

"How did everything go?" my mom asked.

Trying to act as if everything was fine I replied, "So far, so good."

"That's great!" she said with a big smile on her face. "Did you two stop off for lunch?"

"No," said Kathy.

"Good. I want to take you girls out for lunch. Nancy, would you like to go to that little Armenian café that you took me to last time I was out here?" she asked. "I think Kathy would like it, too."

"Sure," I said. "Let's go now."

I picked up David, grabbed his diaper bag and headed for the car. My mom and sister followed.

When we arrived at the restaurant, I was rather quiet during our meal. I tried to engage in some conversation, but found it difficult. All of a sudden, a flood of tears started falling uncontrollably down my face. I quickly grabbed a napkin and wiped my eyes in an effort to prevent my mother from seeing, but it was too late.

"What's the matter, Honey? Why are you crying?" she asked.

"Oh, I'm just stressed out about the offer we made on the house. I wonder if they're going to accept it, and I'm wondering if we're doing the right thing," I said, surprising myself at how quickly I thought up an excuse.

"Don't let that stress you out. You have to take care of yourself," she said.

Hearing her tell me that I had to take care of myself made me feel even more helpless. "Are you going to baby me about everything, and treat me with kid gloves the rest of my life just because I had cancer?" I snapped.

"Honey, I just don't want to see you get so upset over this house. It's not worth it."

"Just leave me alone!" I snapped back again. Nothing was said the remainder of the meal, or during the car ride home.

I dropped my mom and sister off at my brother's house, and then went home to put David down for his nap. I needed to talk to someone. I was unable to reach Kathryn, so I called Laura. Fortunately she was in her office and could spare a few minutes to talk to me. I rehashed everything as she listened.

"Nancy, last time you had an 80-percent chance that it was cancer and a 20-percent chance that it wasn't. This time the odds are the opposite:

Dr. Baick's giving you an 80-percent chance that it's *not* cancer, and a 20-percent chance that it is. I think you're going to be fine," she said.

She had a point. It was easy for everyone to tell me these things, but difficult to believe it. All of the coping mechanisms I used with my cancer diagnosis the first time around went right out the door. It was like hearing that I had cancer for the first time.

About 30 minutes later, my sister walked over from my brother's house. "How are you doing?" she asked.

"Not good," I replied.

"I have something to tell you, and I don't want you to get mad," she said. "Promise?"

"I can't promise anybody anything right now," I snapped back.

"Well, I told Mom."

"You what?" asking for further clarification.

"I told Mom," my sister replied.

"Why did you do that? I specifically told you not to!" I yelled. "You promised."

"I know I broke a promise to you. I admit that, but Mom couldn't understand why you were so rude to her at the restaurant. She asked me if I knew what was going on with you so I told her. Mom's okay. Don't worry. She's glad she knows and I think you're going to feel better, too," she said.

Deep down, part of me did feel better knowing that my mom was aware of the situation. I was glad Kathy told her, because I don't think I could have held out much longer without exploding. "Why don't you walk over to Tod's house and talk to her. I'll stay here with David," she suggested.

"Okay," I said walking out the door.

When I arrived at my brother's house, I knocked on the screen door and walked in. "I heard Kathy told you about the appointment," I said.

"Yes, and I'm glad she did," Mom said, stroking my hair.

We moved over to the couch and sat down. "I'm glad she did, too. I feel better that you know."

"Many women have calcifications appear on their mammograms periodically. Please don't worry. I'm glad Kathy and I will still be here for the procedure. It's a shame we're scheduled to leave the day after the operation. Do you want me to call the airline and change the date?"

"No, that's okay Mom, it's just an outpatient operation," I said. "By the way, I apologize for my behavior at the restaurant. I was just scared and I took it out on you."

"Don't even give it a second thought. There's no need to apologize. I think you've been handling this whole thing extremely well. I don't think I would be able to handle everything as well as you have," she said.

When my brother came home from work that evening, I told him what had happened. I could see in his eyes how badly he felt. "You've been through a lot Nancy, but you are coping so well," he said.

It's nice having Tod live down the street, especially while I was under doctor's care. He was always willing to help us out with David, run errands for us, or just come over to visit and play with David.

Around 7 p.m. that evening, our real estate agent stopped by to tell us that the offer on the house was accepted with a counter offer. The seller wanted a 28-day escrow, as the house would be going into foreclosure. Randy and I agreed that 28 days wasn't ample time to take possession of the property. We already had our 10-day trip to Maui scheduled the first week in April, which would leave us only 18 days to rent or sell our condo, pack our things and move. Moreover, we didn't know the outcome of the biopsy. Based upon the circumstances, it seemed only logical to reject their counter offer. The timing just wasn't right. Again, *everything is as it should be.*

That night I had one less thing to think about as I laid my head down on the pillow. I didn't have to be concerned with the house anymore—just my health. I kept reminding myself that the odds were in my favor that the calcifications would more than likely be benign.

It was still dark outside when Randy and I awoke the next morning at 5:15. Kathy offered to take care of David in the morning so my mom could come to the hospital. It was important for me to have her there. I peeked in David's room to check on him before we left. He was still sound asleep. Just then my mom and sister walked over from my brother's house. Kathy gave me a hug, and wished me good luck. Randy, my mom, and I got into the car and drove to the hospital.

I was beginning to feel as though there was a correlation between my operations, and my mom's visits out to California. Every time I had one, she was there. It never failed—from blood tests to radiation treatments, she was always around to help me with David and to take care of me. I needed my mom now more than ever. We were always close, but after my dad died, we developed an even closer bond.

When we arrived at the hospital, I was given a gown to change into. I was told I could see Randy and my mom prior to going into the operating room, but first I needed to have the needle localization mammogram done. I followed the technician down the hall as Randy and my mom sat in the waiting room.

The technician told me to sit down on the revolving stool in front of the mammogram machine. She began inserting a large needle with a long wire on the end, into my left breast. It was slightly uncomfortable. Dye was then injected into the breast. The wire would remain in my breast during surgery to be used as a guide for Dr. Baick to pinpoint the exact area of tissue to remove. The technician then positioned my breast against the metal plates and took the mammogram.

When that step was completed, I walked back down the hall into the prep room and was told to lie on the gurney. I remember the anesthesiologist, Dr. Botzbach, so well. She was so gentle and kind. Dr. Botzbach told me the types of anesthesia she would be administering, and how I probably wouldn't remember much after we went through the double doors into the operating room. She assured me that everything would be fine, and that she'd be with me the entire time.

"Do you want to see your husband and mom beforehand?" she asked.

"Yes, I was planning on it," I said. One of the attending nurses went out into the waiting room to get them.

"Don't I look cute in this shower cap?" I said facetiously to Randy and my mom, referencing the blue surgical cap on my head.

"You sure do," said Randy giving me a quick peck on the lips. We'll see you when you're out of Recovery.

My mom held my hand and said, "God bless you Honey," as I was wheeled down the hall for surgery.

When I woke up, Dr. Botzbach was beside me. "It's over," she said. "It went really well."

I was fading in and out of consciousness and mumbled a few things about being cold. Within a minute, one of the nurses went to get a blanket out of the blanket warmer and put it over me. I rested for another 20 to 30 minutes before they dressed me and sent me home. I was given instructions not to lift anything over ten pounds for the first three weeks—which included David. I hated having restrictions like that. Every mother wants to be able to hold and lift her child.

After surgery, Dr. Baick told Randy and my mom that I had a 8 a.m. appointment on Thursday to discuss the results of the biopsy. It was yet another period of time to wait out. God, how I hated that! One part of me held on to the 80 percent, which was in my favor. The other part reverted back to the 20 percent, which was not in my favor—someone had to fall into the 20 percent category, it could in fact be me. Then what?

The days leading up to learning the results of the biopsy seemed longer than before. I couldn't help but feel moments of anxiety. I tried to repress my thoughts, but my mind was absorbed by fear; fear of the unknown.

I began talking aloud to God again and prayed that everything would be okay. I couldn't help but wonder why I was being tested. I knew there had to be some message behind all of this, but what was it?

9

Randy took the afternoon off from work to accompany me to Dr. Baick's office for the biopsy results. He could tell I was anxious. I'm sure he was too, although he never let me know it. I think he felt he had to be strong for me so that I wouldn't fall apart, which was a good thing. Had he shown me any signs of fear, I surely would have panicked.

When we arrived, I was greeted by Margo, Dr. Baick's medical assistant. "I know how anxious you must be to get your results," she said. "I'll do my best not to keep you waiting too long." I was grateful for that. Although I had become accustom to waiting days for biopsy results, it didn't make it any less agonizing.

"Randy," I said as we sat in the waiting room, "If I'm diagnosed with cancer, I'm not going to go through radiation therapy again." Although I didn't mean what I had just said, it sure felt good saying it! It gave me a sense of having *some* control! Actually, I would have done whatever Dr. Baick recommended—that's how much I value his opinion. I was nervous and fidgety; I couldn't read any of the magazines. I couldn't do anything except wait to be called.

Finally, Margo said, "Nancy, you can come in now." Randy grabbed my hand and we walked in.

"We haven't received the full report yet," said Margo. "We're waiting for the rest to be faxed to Dr. Baick." Margo took us to a room I had never been in before. It wasn't an examination room like I was usually accustomed to. It was beautiful. *Too* beautiful. There was colorful wallpaper, soft lighting, two lovely couches, and a few attractive chairs. I sensed something was not right. "Margo," I screamed, "This isn't a good a sign!"

"Just sit down and relax. We're still waiting for the fax to come in. Dr. Baick will be in shortly," she said shutting the door behind her. She looked concerned, as though she knew something but was unable to tell me.

We sat down on one of the couches. "Randy," I cried, clutching his hand. "This isn't a good sign! We wouldn't be in this beautiful room unless Dr. Baick had to deliver bad news." My heart was pounding faster and faster. "I can't take anymore!" I cried.

"Get a hold of yourself, Nancy. We still don't know anything yet. Maybe Dr. Baick uses this room to give all women their test results," he said calmly.

"Well, he didn't use it for me last time," I said grabbing a tissue from the box on the table. "See, the room's even prepared with tissue for those who cry!"

Thank God the door opened when it did. God only knew where my mind would have gone next. I was so relieved to see Dr. Baick. He knew not to prolong things with salutations like, "Hi, how are you doing?" He got right down to business, using an old familiar phrase:

"I have some good news and some bad news. The bad news is that it's cancer." Wham! "The good news is that it's the same type of non-invasive cancer you had the first time: Ductal carcinoma in situ. In addition, sections showed marked lobular hyperplasia, a pre-cancer showing no evidence of invasive carcinoma." He walked over to one of the chairs and sat down beside us. "I was very surprised to hear this myself," he said.

Dr. Baick has to deal with telling women this kind of news every day. However, I know it had to be even more difficult with me, as I had already been down this road a little over a year ago. He knew I was a mother of a young baby and what a toll it took on me the first time. Besides, he got to know the sort of person I was—the sort who tends to worry about things before they actually happen.

"I didn't expect this since the odds of this occurring to the opposite breast so quickly are minimal," said Dr. Baick.

"What are her options now?" asked Randy.

"Fortunately the mammogram was able to pick up the microscopic cells. Since it was detected early, you won't need to have an axillary node dissection like you did last time. However, you could do radiation treatments, or have the breast removed." Double wham! I was stunned!

HAVE THE BREAST *REMOVED*!?!

I began crying even harder. I didn't like either of the options, especially having my breast removed! My God! This can't be happening!

"You don't need to make a decision right now," he said.

"We're leaving to go to Hawaii on Sunday," I said wiping my nose. "Do we need to cancel our trip?"

"No, you go and try to enjoy yourselves. Take that time to think about what you want to do," he said.

I've always been the kind of person who has to know what the game plan is from the beginning, and then move forward. I didn't want to mull around for days or weeks dwelling about what I was going to do. I wanted to know what I was going to do right then and there, with Dr. Baick's input.

"If I were your daughter, what would you recommend?" I asked.

"Nancy, you're young, and we all want you to live a long life. You may continue to have similar experiences of abnormalities from time to time throughout your life. I know you don't wish to experience this again. So based upon these reasons, I don't think it's unreasonable for you to consider a double mastectomy."

"A *DOUBLE* MASTECTOMY?!" I screamed. "A minute ago I was just going to lose one breast and now I'm losing two?" The feeling of devastation was overwhelming.

"If you have both of them removed you won't have to worry about having a reoccurrence, and we do elegant reconstruction work."

After I got past the initial shock, I realized Dr. Baick had a good point. If I could have a new occurrence in the opposite breast as quickly as I did, who's to say that I couldn't get a reoccurrence after the radiation therapy?

"What type of implants would you recommend?" I asked.

"For our patients with mastectomies, we recommend silicone. It's much more natural and less apt to deflate over time. I think you'd be happy with them," he said.

"What about the risks associated with silicone implants?" Randy asked.

"We've been using silicone in the body for years. Pacemakers and artificial joints are just a few examples. I think you'll be just fine."

"Will you remove my nipples too?" I asked.

"Yes, we don't want to take any risk of cancer developing in the nipples. The plastic surgeon will use your own skin to reconstruct the nipples for you. Then the areola is tattooed with a darker pigment." (The areola is the circular area around the nipple and is typically darker than the rest of the breast). It was *so* hard to imagine all this.

"Will I have any feeling in my breasts?" I asked.

"You will have some, but not 100 percent," he said.

He then showed us a few snap shots of how reconstructed breasts look. I didn't like what I saw. They didn't look real to me, which only made me feel worse. Dr. Baick sensed my reaction.

"Let us give you a name and phone number of one of our patients who underwent a double mastectomy and reconstruction. She can talk to you and tell you what you can expect," he said. He looked at his nurse

Earlene who was sitting beside him, "Would you mind getting Judy's phone number for Nancy," he asked.

Still feeling extremely nervous and upset about what I had just heard, I asked, "I don't have to undergo chemotherapy, do I?"

"No, you don't. You're cancer is non-invasive," he said. "When are you coming back from your trip?"

"April 15th," Randy responded. "Is it okay if we wait until then?"

"Yes, let's plan on scheduling surgery the week of the 20th. You'll also need to set up a consultation with Dr. Krugman, the plastic surgeon I work with. Earlene will give you his card."

"Is he good?" I asked.

"Yes, all of my patients are very pleased with his work. Call me if you think of any more questions," he said, as he stood up.

Randy shook his hand and thanked him. Earlene gave me Judy's phone number and Dr. Krugman's card.

As we walked out the door, I saw Margo just a few feet away. "I have cancer again," I said in a quivering voice. "I'm going to have a double mastectomy." She reached out and gave me one of the warmest hugs and began crying right along with me. I was so touched by her tenderness. That's one thing I'd have to say about Dr. Baick's staff, they are all so very pleasant and compassionate. He hand-picks the cream of the crop.

Randy and I left Dr. Baick's office, hand in hand. "How does this make you feel?" I asked.

"I'm okay with it as long as you are."

"The fact that I have cancer again came as a surprise. But I have to admit, it wasn't as devastating as hearing it the first time."

"Really?"

"Yes. I guess it's because I'm more educated about breast cancer now. What scared me the most was hearing Dr. Baick say the words *double mastectomy*," I said.

"I can only imagine!" said Randy.

I couldn't wait to get home. I already knew I was going to call my uncle Sam first. He of all people would help me put things into perspective and advise me how I should tell my mom. She was waiting to hear the results—everyone was.

"I'm going to call Uncle Sam," I said as I raced upstairs to our bedroom for privacy.

I called his office and his secretary answered. "Is Dr. Mikaelian available?" I asked.

"He's in a meeting at the moment. May I take a message? "This is his niece calling from California," I said.

Before I could say another word, she said, "Just a minute, I'll get him for you." For years Uncle Sam had advised his secretary to interrupt him during a meeting should anyone from his family call.

A few minutes later I heard his voice on the other end, "Hello."

"Hi Uncle Sam, it's Nancy. I'm sorry to bother you at work but I really need to talk to you. Is this a bad time?" I asked.

"No, Honey, not at all. Did you get the results yet?"

"Yes. It is non-invasive cancer. The same kind I had before," I said crying.

"Okay. What's the treatment this time?"

"Dr. Baick said I could have radiation therapy, but is recommending that I get a double mastectomy to ensure that I live a long life."

"That's not something to get upset about. I know a few women who have had that done and they are very pleased with their results. Get out a piece of paper and let's write down all the positives and negatives no matter how serious or silly they may seem," he said. We took turns rattling things off. By the time we were through, the list looked like this:

PROS	CONS
1) I have LIFE	1) Have to undergo more surgeries
2) It was detected early	2) Will have pain and discomfort
3) Randy is supportive	3) Will have scars, general public won't see
4) Free of fear; peace of mind	4) Will lose some sensation
5) Safer to have another baby	5) Won't be able to breast feed future baby
6) Can choose the size of my breast	
7) Can wear more provocative clothing	
8) Won't have to get my clothes altered	
9) Breasts won't sag when I get older	
10) Won't have to do breast exams	
11) I'll be safer than most women who have breasts	

"Women all over are having breast augmentations. There's probably more women having them out in California anyway, so you'll fit right in," he said.

We both started laughing. I was beginning to feel even better, and more confident about the decision to have the double mastectomy. "Well, now that I mastered that, how on earth am I going to tell my mom about this?" I asked.

"Just like you did last time. You have to be very strong and positive with your delivery. Tell her the results of your biopsy came back positive for cancer and that your doctor recommends you have a double mastectomy. Then go over all of the reasons that we just listed."

"You make it sound so simple," I said.

"You can do it. Make the call now."

"Okay. Thanks for helping me put things into perspective. I love you."

"I love you too, Honey," he said.

I immediately called my mom and got her answering machine. I didn't want to leave a message, so I hung up in despair. I tried to track her down, thinking she may be at my aunt Catherine's house, so I called over there. My aunt answered the phone.

"Hello."

"Aunt Catherine. Hi, this is Nancy."

"Oh, hi Honey, how are you?" she asked with concern.

"By any chance is my mom there?"

"No. She was here this morning and told me about you. Did you get the results of your tests yet?" she asked.

"Yes," I started crying. "It's cancer and I'm having a double mastectomy." She burst out crying, "Oh Honey, I'm so sorry."

"I'll be fine," I said wiping away my tears. "Please don't discuss this with my mom until I get a hold of her."

"You have my word. That needs to come from you," she said. "May God be with you. I love you, Sweetheart."

"I love you, too."

Next I decided to call my sister Kathy and shared the news with her. She didn't handle it well either; she started crying and I ended up consoling her! Then I called my brother Tod. I could tell he felt awful and didn't know what to say—he was speechless. Shortly after I hung up the phone, it rang. It was my mom.

"Hi Honey. I just got in. I decided to call you since there wasn't a message from you on my answering machine."

"I tried calling you," I said, "But I didn't want to leave a message."

"Why? Do you have bad news?" she asked.

"Yes. It's cancer and Dr. Baick is recommending I get a double mastectomy."

"A double mastectomy?" she exclaimed.

"Yes, and here's why." I began to recite the more important reasons off of the positive side of the list that I put together with my uncle. I was able to deliver all of the points clearly and concisely, without shedding a tear.

Nevertheless, she was shocked. She asked me to let her know when the next operation was to be and offered to fly out again and help me. I told her that I didn't know the exact date, but it would probably be the week of April 20th after we returned from Hawaii.

Life is funny. I don't think anyone is ever prepared to handle misfortunes when they occur. However, I have learned that just when you think you can't handle one more thing, another terrible thing comes along just to show you that you can!

Randy knew how much I liked the comedian Adam Sandler, so he suggested we go and see the movie *The Wedding Singer*. "If anyone can make you laugh, I know Adam Sandler can. Let's go—you'll feel better," he said.

I have to admit, as much as I enjoy Adam Sandler's humor, I didn't laugh at all. I was unable to concentrate. I kept thinking about losing my breasts and how badly I wanted this nightmare to end. I'm only in my 30's, I thought. This is suppose to be the best time of my life. I shouldn't be dealing with major things like this at such a young age. As one of my high school friends put it, "That's for old ladies with blue hair not a young mother like you!" More than anything, I wanted to be able to enjoy being a mother and spend time doing things as a family.

When we returned home from the movies, I called a few of my friends to tell them the outcome of the tests I'd just had, and that I was going to have a double mastectomy.

One of my dear friends, Candy, burst into tears. "Nancy, you're one of the nicest people I know. You don't deserve this. You've been through so much with your dad. I don't understand," she said.

Most of my friends cried when I told them. Of course this didn't make me feel any better, but it gave me the opportunity to repeat some of the positive things that were on my list. Once I read those items on the list, my friends began to feel better, and so did I.

Losing both my breasts to cancer wasn't something that I was going to keep a secret nor something that I was going to be ashamed of. This was a time for me to be thankful that the cancer had been detected, and that something could be done. It wasn't all that long ago when being diagnosed with breast cancer was a death sentence.

Things could have been much different had I gotten pregnant *before* the mammogram. Then the cancer would not yet have been detected, and would have festered inside me for nine months, unknown to any of us. Had that been the case, I would have blamed myself for taking the risk to become pregnant. I would have assumed that the female hormones released during pregnancy were the contributing factor causing breast cancer; when in essence, they weren't.

I've never been much of a private person, so I had no qualms about telling everyone I knew that I was going to have a double mastectomy. Even when I had cancer the first time, I grew to be proud to let others know that I was a cancer survivor. Now I was going to be a *two*-time cancer survivor at the age of 37! I wanted people to know that there is a life after cancer.

I wanted spiritual support from everyone—including strangers! I'd tell clerks at department stores and people who were grocery shopping about my cancer. I even went as far as giving homeless people money in exchange for prayers. I felt as though I was an activist on a special quest to rally and support a great cause—my life! The more people I told, the more prayers I would receive. I had spiritual energy flowing from all directions.

Even my travel agent, Jon, put me on prayer chains. I never knew he was such a spiritual man until we began talking about the challenges I was facing. He had connections all over the world. He even had people praying for me in such far away places as England, Canada, and Mexico. The people in those countries would then pass my name and spiritual needs on to others—thus a prayer chain. I was so amazed. Jon asked if he could personally come and pray with me and drop off some literature for me to read after we came back from Hawaii. I welcomed his invitation with open arms.

The following Tuesday I went back to work. I had many things to catch up on. When my boss Rick came into the office, he stopped by my desk and gave me a hug and asked how I was doing. I told him that getting cancer again came as a shock. I laughed and said that I was going to look at this as a boob job instead of a double mastectomy—it's all a matter of semantics. He said it was nice to see what a great attitude I had.

Relocating to a new office building with my part-time position enabled me to meet other associates and develop new friendships. I seemed to bond particularly well with Vicki, who had the nurturing qualities of my own mother.

Vicki has three daughters of her own, one a year younger than me. I always joked around with her and would say she was my surrogate mom. Vicki has a heart of gold—she's a true angel. She was an active philanthropist, volunteering her time and services for several major charitable causes.

I first met Vicki in the ladies room at our offices the first month I started my new job. We began making small-talk, and then I started running in to her more and more. I felt like I had known her for years. She's so warm, friendly, and easy to talk to. I had told Vicki that I was a breast cancer survivor when we first met. She took a special interest in me since two of her sisters and one of her friends were also breast cancer survivors.

I told Vicki about my upcoming surgery, and confided in her the most. I felt comfortable sharing things with her because she gave me the motherly nurturing that I required every day in person, face to face, until my mom arrived. There were some things that I could tell Vicki that I couldn't tell my mom—only because I wanted to spare my mom the worry. Hence, I shared the high highs with my mom, and low lows with Vicki.

Working was actually therapeutic for me. It gave me something else to focus on, as well as an opportunity to pull strength from several of the associates who I had recently met. It seemed everyone had something positive to say, or a success story of some kind to share with me. All of this was very encouraging.

I began counting the days until our trip to Maui, as well as the days to my operation.

10

Before I knew it, we were relaxing on the white sandy beaches of Maui. I tried so hard not to dwell on what was to take place in the weeks ahead. After all, this was our family vacation; a time for rest and relaxation. A time to get away from work and our household stress. A time to pamper ourselves, bask in the sun, snorkel and scuba dive—not a time for me to wallow in self pity and spoil our trip.

Above all, I wanted Randy to enjoy himself; he deserved it. He had been so loving and supportive throughout my breast cancer ordeal. When I told Kathryn how wonderful and accepting he was, she said, "Nancy, not all husbands are like Randy. Some men leave their wives over things like this. They just can't handle it." I never thought about that, but she was right. Whenever I thanked Randy for being there for me, he would always reiterate, "in sickness and in health." He spoke these meaningful, unselfish words straight from the heart.

Our second night in Maui, I woke up at 4 a.m. with a terrible thought. A thought I couldn't let go of. *What if the pathologists detect cancer cells in the breast tissue that is to be removed during the double mastectomy? And, what if those sections of pre-cancer cells that Dr. Baick said were found in the tissue he removed, turned into invasive cancer? Oh God, no! Then I'd have to have chemotherapy!* I tried talking myself out of the crazy hysteria I was entering into, but my mind wouldn't listen.

My thoughts continued...*If I had a 0.8 percent chance per year of getting cancer in the opposite breast, and I got it the following year, anything could happen! Ahhhhhh!!!*

"Randy, Randy," I whispered. "Wake up." "What, what...I'm sleeping."

"I know. I'm sorry to wake you up, but I just had a terrible thought and now I can't sleep." I explained the fearful thought that awoke me from a sound sleep.

"Nancy," he mumbled still half asleep, "The biopsy already showed us that it was the same type of cancer that you had last time. You don't need chemotherapy. Besides, Dr. Baick already removed the breast tissue that contained the cancer. It's no longer in your body. Now go back to sleep and get some rest."

That morning we awoke at 7 a.m., as we had plans to drive the scenic winding *Road to Hana,* which would take three to four hours. Randy sensed I was still preoccupied with my early morning thoughts.

"Nancy, if it's going to make you feel better, call Dr. Baick and have him put your mind at ease."

"That's a great idea," I said grabbing my travel bag looking for my personal address book. "Why didn't I think of that?"

"Because you're too busy thinking about breast cancer," he said jokingly.

I felt a sense of relief just seeing Dr. Baick's name and phone number in my directory. I immediately called his office.

"Is Dr. Baick available?" I asked the receptionist.

"No. He's in surgery. May I take a message?" Damn! Now what? Perhaps his medical assistant Margo would have the answer, I thought.

"Is Margo available?" I asked.

"Yes she is. May I say who's calling?"

"Nancy Madey."

"Please hold."

An instant sigh of relief came over me, as I stood waiting for Margo to come on the line.

"Hello, Nancy. Are you calling from Hawaii?"

"Yes. I'm having a wonderful time so far, except I awoke with this awful thought." I went on to explain my fears.

"I've never heard of anything like that happening before. Can you call back at 2 p.m. when Dr. Baick is out of surgery?"

"I'll make it a point to," I said anxiously.

"Then I'll personally speak with Dr. Baick about your concerns, and have him talk to you when you call back."

"Thanks Margo. I really appreciate it."

Deep down, I was disappointed in myself for having entered into the "what if" game again. It was dangerous, and I knew it. No benefits were to be had. I was only left feeling more afraid than ever—an emotion I could certainly have done without! I realized part of my digression had to with the fact that I was on an island far way from the friends whom I had grown to rely upon for support.

However, we loaded up our rental car and started the drive to Hana. The scenery along the winding roads was so beautiful. We were surrounded by gorgeous green mountains, lush vegetation, and natural water springs. This was truly paradise.

Needless to say, I was preoccupied the entire drive. I kept looking at my watch, waiting for the hours to pass until it was time to call Dr. Baick. Our vacation would have been so much different had I not been going through this terrible experience. I couldn't escape from the dark cloud that lingered over my head.

When we arrived in Hana, we bought some sandwiches and had a little picnic by the ocean. A light misty rain sprinkled across the sunny sky as a beautiful rainbow appeared before our eyes. It was spellbinding!

We took a leisurely drive around the town of Hana before heading back to our hotel. Along the way we came upon a beautiful waterfall. We pulled off to the side of the road to get a closer look. In the distance, I noticed a telephone.

"Randy, I see a phone! I'm going to call Dr. Baick now," I said running toward the telephone. I anxiously pulled my calling card out of my wallet, and began punching the telephone number into the phone.

"Comprehensive Breast Health Center. May I help you?" the voice on the other end answered.

"Yes. This is Nancy Madey calling from Hawaii. Dr. Baick is expecting my call," I said nervously.

"One moment Nancy. Let me connect you."

Within seconds Dr. Baick was on the phone, "Nancy, you're supposed to be enjoying your vacation!"

"I know Dr. Baick, but I got scared and needed to call you for clarification. Did Margo tell you my concerns?" I asked.

"Yes, and the odds of additional cancer cells being found in the breast tissue that's to be removed during the mastectomy are extremely rare. Please try and enjoy your vacation, and don't worry about things like that," he said. Just hearing his reassuring voice was all that I needed to mentally get me through the rest of our vacation. I felt like a new person when I hung up the phone.

I ran over to Randy who was watching the waterfall with David. "Randy," I yelled waving my hands. "I don't need to worry anymore!" Randy was thrilled to see me happy and smiling again.

On our anniversary, we drove to the other side of the island and found a beautiful beach and relaxed in the sun. Afterward, Randy took me shopping and bought me a lovely dress and some Hawaiian perfume. We ended the evening at a fancy restaurant on the ocean—it was as romantic as we could get with little David there, but we wouldn't have had it any other way.

Suddenly, the vacation was over. I was actually looking forward to going home and preparing for the next event. I still had to set up an appointment for the consultation with Dr. Krugman, finalize a surgery date, and then get mentally, spiritually and emotionally prepared to have the double mastectomy.

When we got home, I unpacked my things and checked our answering machine for messages. Dr. Baick's office had called saying the surgery date was scheduled for Friday, April 24th at 1 p.m., and the procedure would take approximately four hours.

The next day, I called Dr. Krugman's office, and set up the consultation for Wednesday, April 15th at 3 p.m. That evening, Randy and I sat down and composed a two-page list of questions to ask Dr. Krugman—everything from what the procedure would involve, down to size of the implants he would recommend.

I also called Judy, the patient Dr. Baick had referred me to, and told her I'd be undergoing a double mastectomy in less than two weeks. While speaking with Judy, I could understand why Dr. Baick suggested I call her. She was so positive, happy, and thrilled with her new breasts. This confirmed that I was doing the right thing. Judy had had the same type of cancer as I did, ductal carcinoma in situ, but only in one of her breasts. She could have had a lumpectomy followed by radiation like I did, but she opted to give up *both* breasts instead. In retrospect, I wish I had done the same the first time, but I didn't expect to develop cancer in the opposite breast, especially so soon after.

I told her I had seen a few snapshots that Dr. Baick had shown me, and how disappointed I was with what I saw. "Those snap shots don't do justice," she said. "I'll be more than happy to show my breasts to you before your operation. That way you can see for yourself just how real they look," she said.

"Would you mind?" I asked.

"Not at all," said Judy. "I do this all the time for women who are going through this. I think it's very important for you to know what to expect."

I spoke with Judy for well over an hour. I felt as though I had known her for years. Her voice was so soothing and energetic. Most of all, she was extremely positive and cheerful. Every time I posed a fear or negative concern, she would turn it into something positive.

"Nancy," Judy said, "this is a time of jubilation for you. How wonderful that the breast cancer was detected so early. Look at all of the rewards: you'll be cancer-free and you'll never have to worry about this again," she said.

And, when I spoke to her about the loss of breast sensation, she replied, "What you lose in sensitivity you'll gain in femininity." What a beautiful thought!

Judy said she had initially opted for saline implants. "One morning I woke up and my left side was deflated," she said laughing. "After that I decided to try the silicone implants. There's no comparison. I'm so much happier and they feel more life-like."

I was looking forward to meeting Judy. She even gave me her business phone number and said she was honored to help me. Can you imagine that? Honored to help me! A complete stranger! She was angelic. "You can call me anytime," she said. After speaking with her, I felt as though I was operating from a position of power rather than a position fear.

"I hope that one day I can be like you," I said.

"Oh, and you will. You'll be helping people just like yourself when you're through," she said. "It helps so much to talk to someone who's already been down that road. I'll walk you through each stage of your reconstructive process. I believe that people need others not only to hold their hand, but to hold their heart too," she said compassionately.

"Thank you so much for taking the time to talk with me. I feel better already.

"It's truly my pleasure," she said.

I felt so blessed to have someone like Judy in my life. Someone who not only had been through the process, but someone who could add the positive influence I so badly needed.

The next day I called Judy from work to thank her again for all her help. During our conversation she said she had some free time over her lunch hour and would be more than happy to meet me somewhere and show me her breasts. I'm sure that would sound rather odd to someone who wasn't in our shoes! We decided to meet at a local fast food restaurant. We described ourselves to each other, as well as what we were wearing, so we would recognize one another.

I arrived at the restaurant earlier than expected. I sat down in one of the booths looking for a blonde woman in her mid-50's, wearing an olive green pantsuit. A few minutes later I noticed a stunningly attractive woman fitting her description, however she looked at least 15 years younger—she just radiated. It has to be Judy, I thought.

"Judy?" I asked.

"Yes, and you must be Nancy," she said extending her hand with a warm smile.

"It's so nice to meet you," I said. "I really appreciate you doing this for me. I just don't know what to expect the finished product to actually look like."

"I think you'll be pleasantly surprised."

Judy motioned for me to walk into the ladies room, so I followed. I felt rather strange and uncomfortable at first, and was thankful that no one else was in the restroom. We both entered a large stall and Judy unbuttoned her blouse to reveal her breasts to me. I was totally amazed.

Stunned, actually. They were *perfect*.

"These are reconstructed?" I asked. "They look unbelievably real."

"Don't they? I'm just thrilled. I decided to go bigger than before. Now I'm able to have fun wearing all sorts of clothes that I wasn't able to wear before because my breasts were smaller."

"Where are your scars?" I asked, as I didn't see an indication of any incisions. She pointed to the top portion of her breast, "Right here. It's been over five years so all of my scars have faded. In time, yours will, too."

I was curious and wondered how they felt to the human touch. "This may sound forward, and I can understand if you say no, but may I just touch one of your breasts just to see what it feels like?"

"Absolutely. It's important for you to know."

I timidly extended my index finger and gently pushed down on the upper portion of her breast. "It feels like breast tissue," I said. "And your nipples look so real. I would have never known they weren't real if you didn't tell me."

"Dr. Baick and Dr. Krugman are the best," she said buttoning up her blouse. "The two of them are a great team."

"I haven't met Dr. Krugman yet. I have a consultation with him tomorrow," I said.

"Trust me. You're in really good hands. Dr. Baick wouldn't work with just anyone. He's extremely particular about only working with the best. He wants his patients to be happy with their results."

I offered to buy her lunch and she refused. "It's my birthday today and I have plans with the folks in my office."

"Well happy birthday! You certainly are one special lady to meet me here on your birthday."

"Oh, it's nothing," she said. "Stay in touch."

"I will."

I felt so much better. I couldn't wait to go back to work and tell Kathryn and Vicki what I did over my lunch hour. They were pleased that I felt so much better, and agreed that it takes a special person like Judy to be able to do something like that.

That evening Randy was delighted to see how happy I was after my meeting with Judy. He too, was very thankful for what Judy had done for me.

In the meantime, I kept mentally conditioning myself that I was having a boob job, not a double mastectomy. Thinking along those lines helped me to focus more on the cosmetic aspects, as opposed to what the cancer was actually stripping me of. I was beginning to feel overjoyed about getting larger breasts and being able to buy new clothes—what woman wouldn't?

The next morning I made plans to carpool to work with Tod so Randy and I could drive together to Dr. Krugman's office. I was anxious to have the consultation with Dr. Krugman, as he was the person responsible for rebuilding my breasts. I was excited to learn about the process and what I could expect.

Shortly after Randy and I arrived, I was called in and we were lead to an examination room. Randy and I waited until Dr. Krugman entered the room.

"Hello. I'm Dr. Krugman, and this is my medical assistant, Laurie," he said.

"It's nice to meet you. This is my husband, Randy."

"Dr. Baick has already gone over your history with me, so I'm aware that you've undergone radiation therapy. To be frank with you," he said, "I have had only one patient who had radiation prior to breast reconstruction. All of the women who I have performed breast reconstructions on, with the exception of one, have chosen to get their breasts removed from the very beginning. But, I understand that you're situation is rather unique. I have to tell you that there *are* risks involved," he said. Once again, I felt my heart sink.

"What are the risk factors," I asked in a concerned manner.

"Radiation knocks off the blood supply creating a loss of expansion. You're breasts may be more prone to encapsulate as well," he said.

I was unfamiliar with the terms *encapsulate* and *expand*, so he defined them for me.

"*Encapsulation* is a formation of a capsule around a structure. In this case it would be the implant. Hard capsules can form around the implant, causing the breast to become extremely firm and sometimes painful, and often requiring the surgical removal of the implant. In some cases, we may take tissue from other areas of the body like the abdomen, to build the breast. But looking at you, you don't have an ounce of fat to spare. In which case, we'd take it from behind your shoulder and move it around to the front of your breast." None of this sounded good. I tried to erase it from my mind and continued listening.

"When I talk about *expansion*, I'm referring to the elasticity of your skin. Dr. Baick and I will both be in the operating room, working in tandem. He will remove the breast tissue and when he's finished, I will begin the immediate first-stage reconstruction. After your mastectomy, a temporary expander will be surgically inserted. The expander has a valve in which we are able to inject saline on a weekly basis. Once you're comfortable with the size, we'll arrange for your Stage 2 reconstruction," he said.

"What does Stage 2 reconstruction involve?" I asked.

"That would involve removing the expanders and replacing them with implants. Stage 3 will be the nipple-areola reconstruction. Laurie can show you a sample of the expander after our consultation," he said.

"I was just looking at this as a breast augmentation to help me deal with it better," I said.

"Oh no. This is much more involved than that. But do whatever you need to do to help you deal with it," he said.

Then I handed him my two-page printout of questions. "This is a good idea," he said. "Are you a school teacher?" he asked.

"No, why?"

"You're just so organized. I've never had a patient do this for me before. I like it. Let's just run down your list," he said.

He read each question aloud and answered it. I also had a copy in my hand so I wrote his answer beneath each of the questions. Some of the more important questions were:

1) Where will the new scar locations be?
2) Since I had an axillary node dissection on my right side, will that create any complication during surgery? Will I be more prone to infection?
3) Do you recommend silicone or saline implants?
4) How long do the implants last?
5) How much sensation can I expect?
6) Are there any possible problems down the road (punctures, leaks, etc.)? If so, what could it do to me?
7) How long will the entire process take from start to finish?
8) How long will the first, second and third surgeries last?

I was distressed to learn that the entire reconstruction process could take anywhere from nine months to one year. He kept assuring me that the slower we'd go, the more pleased I'd be with the final results.

After our consultation, Laurie showed us an expander. It looked like a small round deflated ball, the size of a grapefruit. She picked up the expander to demonstrate its flexibility by squeezing it a few times, and then handed it to me. Although it was silicone, its outside texture wasn't smooth. It was rather grainy, with a metal valve attached to one side. She explained the expansion process and how most of their patients begin expanding two to three weeks after surgery. Then she took two Polaroid snapshots of my breasts for the files.

On the way home I started crying. Hearing all of the risks associated with the radiation really frightened me. For an instant, I even entertained the idea of not having reconstructive surgery—anything to avoid the potential risks. I was beginning to feel depressed and was running out of options.

"Nine months to one year" kept echoing inside my head. Cancer had already consumed one year of my life. Now it's going to take yet another, I thought.

Having to wait another year also meant that we'd have to postpone trying to have a baby until the spring of 1999. I'd be 38 years old, and 39 by the time I gave birth.

What if I didn't get pregnant as quickly as I did with David? It would also mean that our children would be four years apart, and I wanted them to be closer in age. I felt as though I was being robbed of making choices in my life: Everything was being predetermined for me, based on the fact that I had cancer. Not once, but twice!

I reflected back on my dad's experience with cancer, recalling how he faced his fears. He had courage, strength and determination, and I knew I needed to have the same. I needed to face the fear, too!

This was the hand I was dealt. Of course, I didn't like it—who would? But I was determined not to let myself fail. I couldn't. I needed to be a wife to Randy and a mother to our son.

I knew I couldn't change reality, but I could change my attitude. I could choose to be angry and feel depressed, or I could accept the situation and go on living my life the best I could. I chose the latter.

The next day at work I received a phone call from David, the president of the company. He mentioned that my brother Tod (also an employee) had stopped by his office to tell him about my most recent diagnosis. I was surprised Tod told David, but knew he would have only told him with my best interest in mind. Tod knew that David was very concerned about my situation when I was diagnosed with breast cancer the first time, and how much better I felt after speaking to him. I had plans to eventually tell David of the new developments, but hadn't brought myself around to doing so.

David asked me if I had some free time to meet with him. Naturally, I made myself available. I knew I would feel better after talking to David, he just had that kind of affect on people.

When I reached the executive offices, his secretary told me to go right in, as David was expecting me. His door was open, and I saw him sitting at his desk, working. I knocked on the door as I slowly entered his office. He looked up and immediately put down his pen.

"Well come on in," he said standing up to greet me. "Thank you for taking the time to speak with me," I said.

"Don't mention it. Let's sit down over here," he said walking over to the opposite end of his office where there was a meeting table, a couch, and a few chairs. "Please, sit down," he said pointing to the couch. He sat in the chair beside me.

"Tod filled me in. He told me you were having a difficult time, which is totally understandable. So bring me up to speed and tell me what's been going on."

He listened closely as I summarized everything that had happened, from the time Dr. Baick found the micro-calcifications on my mammogram, to the consultation I just had with Dr. Krugman.

We talked openly and frankly about my double mastectomy. He told me that I needed to take time and put things into perspective. "You're going to be prolonging your life. Granted, having this series of surgeries will be not be pleasant, but you can't lose sight of the reason why you're doing this," he said.

He continued to counsel me as I sat and absorbed every word he said. When we finished talking, he gave me a big, long hug.

"If there's anything you need, or anything I can do to help you out, please call me. I want to hear how you're progressing. I know you're going to do just fine, Sunshine," he said.

That afternoon, I had the final consultation with Dr. Baick about the double mastectomy. I told him how fearful I had become after Dr. Krugman outlined the risks.

"Did Dr. Krugman feel your radiated breast?" he asked. "No," I replied.

"Perhaps that's why. Your breast responded well to the radiation. Most women's breasts get extremely hard," he said. "I'm sure if Dr. Krugman had felt it, he would have been pleased by the lack of hardness. You have a good success rate, Nancy. Don't worry."

Dr. Baick removed all of my fears. I had my confidence back and I was ready to have the operation right then and there. I didn't think I could last another week.

The following week, my friend Jon called to see if he could stop by that evening and do some spiritual meditation with me. I was open to anyone who was willing to provide me with any form of positive reinforcement.

When he arrived, we chatted and reminisced about our days together in travel school. I also told him that today, April 21, 1998, was the four-year anniversary of my father's death. Jon was aware that my dad and I had a very close relationship and wished he had had the opportunity to know him.

"I'm glad you shared that with me Nancy, because I'd like to bring your father into our meditation process," he said in his English accent. "Are you ready to get started?" he asked.

"Yes," I said, not knowing what to expect. He pulled out one of our dining room chairs and turned the back of the chair so it was facing the table. Then he pulled out another one of our dining room chairs and placed it across from me. We were now sitting face to face.

"Close your eyes," he said. "Now breathe slowly in and out."

I did exactly what he said. "Very good. Now try to focus on finding a white Light in the center of your being." He explained the Light was God, the Holy Spirit.

I waited for a white Light to appear, but nothing happened. "Jon, I don't see anything," I said.

"Be patient, it will come." Still nothing. As he talked more about finding this soft white Light, the healing Light, I expected to miraculously see it. Still nothing. I was beginning to feel frustrated, so he made a suggestion.

"We'll try something different," he said. "When I close my eyes, I am able to see the white Light. Let me hold your hands, so that the energy of the healing Light will flow through my hands into yours."

I gave Jon my hands and he held them firmly. He began praying to God. He asked God to cleanse my body of any and all cancer cells that may remain, and to generate new healthy cells in their place.

All of a sudden I felt a surge of energy. "Jon!," I exclaimed in a low voice, "I'm feeling a warm tingling sensation entering my body from the ground. It's starting at the bottom of my feet, now it's traveling up to my knees, and now it's surging through my arms!" I exclaimed with my eyes closed. "Now I see the Light, Jon, I see the Light!" I exclaimed again.

"That's wonderful. Let the Light guide you," he whispered softly. "Let God touch every cell in your body."

Jon continued talking to me and praying over my body. I heard him stand up as he walked behind my chair and placed his hands over my head. The more he prayed over me, the more relaxed and at peace I became. He even spoke to my dad, bringing him into the script. Although my eyes were closed, tears were falling down my face. Jon gently wiped each tear away. The entire experience lasted about 10 or 15 minutes. I was amazed to think that God was working inside me. Then, he told me to slowly open my eyes.

When I awoke, I felt refreshed, alert, and alive. I felt as though I had slept for ten hours, although I knew that no more than 15 minutes had passed. I felt stripped of all negative concepts. I had no fear. I felt inner peace. I felt strong enough to move mountains. In essence, *I Let Go and Let God* take over. It was amazing how great I felt. I knew I had just had another religious experience.

I thanked Jon and marveled over what I had just experienced. He offered to come over the morning of my operation to pray with me again. How could I refuse? It would be wonderful if I could feel like this the day of my surgery, I thought.

That night I slept like a baby. My mind was totally at peace. I was surprised to discover that I felt just as good the next morning when I awoke.

When I arrived at work, I told Kathryn and Vicki about my religious experience with Jon. They could actually see in my face and hear in my voice that I was a changed woman. It was obvious to both of them that something wonderful had happened.

I continued getting support from all of my friends and family up to the date of the operation. Vicki and Kathryn would always check in with me to make sure my spirits were still high.

Earlier in the week, Vicki introduced me to a woman who's office was near Vicki's. Her name also was Judy. Judy was active in volunteering her services for the American Cancer Society—breast cancer in particular. She offered to provide me with literature, and said that if I ever needed anything to please let her know. She said she was impressed by how well composed I was.

"I don't think I would be as strong as you," she said. "Especially at your young age." I loved getting compliments like that—it was so encouraging, and made me feel even stronger.

The day before my operation, Vicki and Judy stopped by my office to wish me well.

"We thought you'd like a little something to hug and keep you company after your surgery," said Vicki. "So, we got you this..." She pulled out an adorable soft, fuzzy lion.

"And, so your son won't get jealous and take it away," Judy said, "We got him this..." She pulled out a white and brown cuddly dog.

"Boy, you guys think of everything," I said. "Thank you so much." I gave them each a hug and they said they'd pray for me. "I'll have my husband or my mom call you after the surgery to let you know that I'm okay. And, I will be okay," I said.

By the end of the day, I had received several phone calls and warm wishes from my associates. I'd tell them that in six weeks, when I came back, they were going to see a new and improved me.

My mom had already been in town for two days. It was comforting for me to have her by my side as I faced the weeks ahead. Everyone had called to wish me well before my operation, including Father Yeprem and Pastor Tim. Those I talked to commented on my sense of calmness and inner peace. "I attribute it all to God," I'd say. "I know He'll take care of me because I'm in a safe place—His hands."

11

It was Friday, April 24, 1998. It was going to be a day I'd never forget. I'd be undergoing a double mastectomy at the young age of 37. Although I'd be losing both breasts, I chose to focus on losing the cancer. I didn't bother worrying about what I was going to look like without breasts, how I would feel, or how my husband would react. I just wanted the cancer *out* of my body. I didn't have the mental capacity to think about anything else.

When I awoke that morning, I made a conscious decision *not* to look at my breasts—not in the mirror, not in the shower and not while drying myself off. I didn't want to be reminded of what I was about to lose forever. I replaced the thought of losing my breasts with a vision of how wonderful the new breasts would be.

The operation was scheduled for 1 p.m.; however, I was told to be at the hospital by 11 a.m. to prepare for surgery. The operation was expected to last approximately four hours.

Jon came over at 9:30 a.m. to pray with me again privately. This time, my experience was drastically different. I didn't feel as energized as I did the first time. The experience was more emotional. I shed more tears, yet remained composed. Before leaving, we all made a circle and held hands; Jon, Randy who was carrying David, my mom, our baby sitter, and me. Jon lead us in a beautiful prayer and then wished me well before he left.

At 10:30 a.m., my mom, Randy and I left to go to the hospital. When we arrived, we all sat quietly waiting. Within ten minutes, I was called in. The nurse said that my husband and mother could come in and see me once I was prepped.

I was given a large plastic bag to store my shoes and clothing in, and then handed a gown and told to get undressed. Afterward, I was lead to a gurney and asked to lie down.

A nurse took my blood pressure and temperature—everything was normal. Next she inserted a needle into the top of my wrist to start the I.V. It was very uncomfortable. She told me she was having problems advancing the needle into the vein. The more she struggled with the needle, the more excruciating the pain. She continued forcing the needle into my wrist. I turned my head in the opposite direction, clenched my teeth and began cringing with pain. "We may have to start all over," she said.

"No, please no," I pleaded. "I can't go through this pain again." I tried my best to stay calm while she continued prodding the needle into my wrist. It was extremely important for me to stay calm so I could enter the operating room in good spirits. Yet, somehow I felt the nurse was gradually stripping me of all my fortitude—the energy I needed to maintain my inner peace.

"I don't understand why the I.V. isn't working," she said. No sooner after she finished her last sentence she exclaimed, "Oh wow, look at that! The I.V. is dripping now. I don't believe it."

Tears of joy streamed down my face. At that moment, I knew it was the work of God. Now, I could go into the operating room with a sense of security. God was with me and so was my guardian angel, my dad.

Soon after, my mom and Randy came in. I told them what had just miraculously happened. Before either of them could respond, the anesthesiologist, Dr. Botzbach, entered the room. I was extremely happy to see her, as I specifically requested to have Dr. Botzbach, although there was no guarantee. Therefore, I was doubly pleased when she came in. Just another positive sign from God, I thought. Dr. Botzbach remembered me from the previous biopsy and was sorry to hear that I was having to undergo a double mastectomy.

To my surprise, my brother stopped by during his lunch hour to wish me well. "You look so calm and composed," he said.

"I am. I'm more than ready to have this operation," I said. "I've been counting the days."

Dr. Baick came in next. Now the room was getting full. I loved being surrounded by everyone, and drew strength from those who were with me. "How are you doing?" he asked with a smile.

"I'm doing great. But most important of all, I'm in a good frame of mind," I boasted.

"That certainly helps," he said. He reviewed the amount of time I'd be in surgery as Dr. Botzbach began injecting the drugs into the I.V. She said she'd be with me the entire time. She explained that a tube would be inserted into my mouth to help me breathe, as this was a general anesthetic and I would not be breathing on my own.

It was now time to begin the operation. I said goodbye to Randy, my mom and Tod as I was wheeled away on the gurney into the operating room.

When I awoke after surgery, I recall looking at the clock. It was 5:15 p.m. I closed my eyes, remembering the reason I was in the hospital. My first thought was how thankful I was to be 100 percent cancer-free—not that I just lost two breasts. While in recovery, I asked Dr. Botzbach if the clock was right. She said it was and that the doctors finished ahead of schedule.

About an hour after recovery, I was wheeled on the gurney to a hospital room on the fourth floor. I vaguely remember seeing Randy and my mom in the elevator, but had no energy to talk.

When in the hospital room, I heard other voices. The voices were my sister-in-law Daryl and Randy's cousin Paul, making small talk with my husband and mom. I was extremely groggy the remainder of the night and just slept.

The next morning when I awoke, I noticed that the room was filled with flowers, plants and balloons. It truly helped to create a cheery atmosphere. I continued to sleep off and on until I heard someone walk into the room. I opened my eyes and was surprised to see Randy's bright, cheerful face. He had a beautiful bouquet of flowers in his hands. "These are for you."

"They're gorgeous. Thank you."

"How are you feeling?" he asked, sitting down at the bedside.

"Not bad. I managed to take a few steps to the bathroom this morning," I said. "And it sure wasn't easy having to wheel this I.V. pole around with me."

"Are you in any pain?"

"No. I've been pumped up with so many drugs that I don't feel a thing. It's just uncomfortable having all of this tubing on me," I said, making reference to the I.V. and drains. "By the way, what did the doctors say?"

"They said that everything went well. You actually were out of surgery 30 minutes ahead of time," he said, grabbing my hand. "You look good, Honey."

"Oh, come on...How's David?"

"He's doing fine. Your mom's watching him. He was asking for you this morning."

"Don't tell me that, it breaks my heart! I miss that little guy," I said smiling.

Just then one of the nurses came in and told me that Dr. Krugman would be making the rounds soon and needed to see me before I could be released.

There's no way that I'm going to be released today, I thought. That's unheard of. Randy read the newspaper and drank a cup of coffee while I closed my eyes and rested. I awoke when I heard Dr. Krugman's voice in the corridor.

"How are you doing?" he asked as he entered the hospital room.

"Pretty good. I'm just sleepy."

"Well, before I release you to go home, I want you to eat something."

"I don't think I'm ready to go home. And, I'm certainly not hungry," I said.

"I'll give you a few more drugs to boost you up. You'll have an appetite and will be surprised at how good you'll feel. You'll want to go home after that," he said. "Anyway, the surgery went well. However, during surgery I noticed that most of your muscle was destroyed on the radiated breast, just as I expected."

"Is that something to be concerned about?" I asked.

"Well, I'll just have to be extra careful as we move forward," he said jotting down a few notes.

"When can I expect to get the pathology report?" I asked.

"You'll have to check with Dr. Baick's office. Usually it's about four days. I'm sure you'll be fine, and once you know for sure you'll feel even better."

"I sure will," I said.

"The nurse will give you instructions about how to empty your drains when you sign all of the release papers. I'll see you in my office on Tuesday, April 28," he said.

Randy and I thanked him as he left. Within minutes, the nurses came to inject the drugs that were to boost me up and give me an appetite. Before I knew it, I was feeling much better and was ready to eat the soup, chicken and green beans that were set before me.

An hour later the nurse came by with the release papers. She went over the instructions for me to follow at home, as well as how to care for the drains that I had on each side. Since I had had a drain with my axillary node dissection, I was familiar with what I needed to do.

"An orderly will be right up with your wheelchair and then you can go home," said the nurse.

"I can't believe how incredibly fast those drugs worked. I would have never thought I'd be able to eat, let alone go home."

"Seeing is believing," he said.

Randy gathered my things as we waited for the orderly. When she arrived, she carefully helped me get into the wheelchair and wheeled me out to our car. Randy carefully helped me get situated in the front seat, and then put a seat belt around me. I was excited to go home and see little David.

When we drove up to the front of our house, a few of our neighbors were sitting outside with my mom, who was playing with David. My neighbors, as well as my mother, were amazed to see how mobile I was. I may have been walking rather slowly and hunched over, but nonetheless, I was moving!

My neighbor, Dean, said, "Man, Nancy. You sure are brave. I don't think I could be as courageous as you." Hearing that comment from a man carried even more weight. It really made me feel good.

My mom picked up David and held him up near me. "Here's mama," she said holding him up to me so I could kiss him.

"Mama's back—I love you so much," I said giving him a kiss. I so badly wished that I could wrap my arms around him and smother him with even more kisses.

Once in the house, Randy helped me to get comfortable on the couch. My mom sat down on the chair beside me and we talked. I told her how wonderful I felt knowing that I'm cancer-free and I don't have to worry about this awful disease anymore.

"I can't believe that you're up and around after seeing you yesterday," she said.

"It is amazing, isn't it? Did you call everyone in Wisconsin to let them know I'm alright?" I asked.

"Yes, I told them that you made it through surgery with flying colors." A few hours later I called several of my friends to let them know I was doing fine. They couldn't believe how well I sounded and that I was even able to make a phone call. I took it easy and rested the remainder of the day and night.

The next day was a different story. I felt like a Mack truck literally ran across my chest. I felt so stiff and sore. I couldn't even get out of bed by myself. Randy tried to help me, but was initially unsuccessful. He was unable to pull me up by the arms because that would strain my chest muscles. Then we finally discovered a way. He placed his open hand behind my neck and gradually raised my upper torso into a sitting position. From there, I was able to swing both legs over the side of the bed and stand up with his assistance. I was totally dependent on Randy and my mother to get me out of bed. In fact, we actually hooked up baby monitors in our bedroom upstairs as well as our kitchen. That way if I needed something, I could be heard downstairs.

I was faithful about taking the prescription of Vicodin every four hours around the clock, as well as measuring and logging the amount of fluid I was collecting in each drain.

When I went to see Dr. Krugman on Tuesday for my post-op appointment, he said I was progressing nicely. However, I needed to keep the drains in. He asked to see me again on Friday.

Later that afternoon Dr. Baick's office called to tell me that the pathology report came back. Everything was fine. No cancer cells were found in the breast tissue that was removed. I was overjoyed. It's always easy to assume that things are going to be OK, but actually *knowing* that they are makes a world of difference.

After my experience with breast cancer, I came to the realization that I was not as invincible as I once thought. If I can fall into categories where

I'm the *one* in 622 women at the age of 35 to develop breast cancer, as well as fall into the 0.8 percent category of women who develop cancer in the opposite breast the following year, then anything can happen.

I began to keep a personal journal of my experience after the mastectomy. I found it very therapeutic to write down my thoughts and feelings. In addition, Randy and I kept a baby journal for David. In fact, we started it when I was pregnant with him. We'd write about our joys of becoming new parents, visits to the obstetrician, feeling his first movements, etc. We continued to write in his journal even after he was born; it was an extension of his baby book. Randy and I would write down funny things David would say or do, as well as share our thoughts and feelings about him, and the things that were going on in our family. This is an excerpt from an entry I wrote in David's baby journal shortly after the double mastectomy:

Wednesday, April 29, 1998

Well, I had the surgery five days ago and everyone is amazed at how well I'm doing. I only had a few days of pain and discomfort.

My attitude is superior, if I must say so myself. Yesterday, I found out that all of the tissue that was removed from both breasts did not contain one cancer cell. The best news is that I will not need any radiation or chemotherapy.

David, I learned so much through this experience. The good Lord is always there for you and you must always give thanks and call upon Him. He loves you and will protect you. Faith in Him removes all fear. By turning all of your fears over to God, you are left with inner peace and a renewed strength. I have a wonderful new relationship with God that I would not have had otherwise.

The operation (approximately 4 hours long) was a success, and miracles are happening everyday. When you get old enough to understand, I want to be able to share all of the joys of this experience with you. In a time of crisis, it's important for a person to face his/her fears—not run from them.

I have a feeling you know what's going on—you want me to lift you up and I can't—doctor's orders for several months. I kneel down, hug and kiss you and scratch your back a lot—you love that! Grandma Mikaelian is here helping, so you're getting lots of love and attention. We all love you, and you are an integral part of my healing process. Just listening to you giggle and play, and seeing you smile is all the medicine I need.

I'm 100-percent cancer-free, and it feels so good to know that I'll be here for you and Daddy. Praise God!

On Friday I went to see Dr. Krugman again. I couldn't believe how fast the first week went by. I explained that I could feel the expanders inside me and how much they hurt, especially when I sneezed. I was told that once the expanders were injected with saline and inflated, it would relieve the pressure I was experiencing.

"You're still draining a lot of fluid," he said. "I'm sorry to disappoint you, but we won't be removing your drains today," said Dr. Krugman.

I was indeed disappointed. I was getting sick and tired of having all of those tubes dangling from my sides and having to measure, and log the drainage two to three times a day. Dr. Krugman wanted to see me again on Tuesday, May 5. I was hopeful the drains would be removed then.

Unfortunately, they still weren't ready to come out as I was continuing to drain fluid. He wanted to see me again in two more days. Hopefully, the drains would be removed then, I thought.

The routine of draining, measuring, and logging the amount of fluid was getting really old by this time. I was sick of the morning sponge bath routine. I was sick of washing my hair over the sink. I was sick of wearing big baggy clothes to conceal all of the apparatus. I was sick of everything. I just wanted to move on to the expansion process.

Several arrangements of flowers and gifts were being delivered to our house on a daily basis. The mailbox was overflowing with stacks of get well cards. It was so nice knowing that I was cared about. I felt blessed to have such wonderful people in my life, and at the same time, thought how difficult it must be for those who do not.

For several days I felt tempted to peek underneath the gauze bandages, but I never did. Part of me was curious to see what I looked like, and the other part was apprehensive. I was afraid of how I would react to seeing myself without any breasts, and without any nipples. I imagined it would be a pretty scary sight. I knew sooner or later I'd have to step up to the plate and look at myself, but I didn't know when that day would be.

One day shy of two weeks, the drains and stitches were removed. At last, true freedom! Dr. Krugman said I could begin the expansion process the next week. That was encouraging—I began to feel I was making progress.

Then one day, my attention began to draw away from myself as I noticed how quiet and depressed Randy had become. My mom noticed the change in him, too. I knew there could only be one reason for this odd behavior—it was obviously because of my situation. Not only was his wife going through major changes, he was too.

Perhaps I made a mistake, I thought. I shouldn't have had Randy in the examination room when the nurse removed the drains and stitches. That's when Randy saw me without breasts and without nipples for the first time. I'm sure that had to be it—it must have had a terrible impact on him. I'm sure it wasn't easy for him to see me so disfigured.

I decided to call Judy, the woman who showed me her reconstructed breasts, to update her on my situation. I told her that the stitches and drains were removed.

"Just wait until you start the expansion process," she said. "It's amazing to see your chest grow before your own eyes."

"I can't wait," I said. "I'm going to start it next week." "That's so exciting," she said.

I also told her about Randy's recent mood changes.

"That's totally understandable," she said. "This man loves you— you're his wife. He has no idea what to expect. You do, because I showed you. If you want, I can stop by your house later this evening and show my breasts to both him and your mother," she said sweetly.

"You'd do that for me?" I asked.

"Of course. I think it's important for both of them. I don't want your mother to have to go back to Wisconsin and worry about what her daughter's going to look like. And, I certainly don't want Randy to continue worrying about what his wife is going to look like. This way they'll both know what to expect."

"You are such an angel," I said. I gave her directions to our house and she said she'd be over after 6:30 p.m.

I told my mom exactly what Judy said and how she offered to come over to our house tonight and show her and Randy.

"I think Judy's right," my mom said. "You are so fortunate to have her help you, Nancy. She sounds like a wonderful woman."

"She is Mom, just wait until you meet her," I said.

I called Randy at work and told him that I had spoken to Judy, who offered to come by that evening and show her breasts to him and my mother. I explained how important I thought it was for him to see the end results. He agreed.

Later that evening, Judy came over. Randy wasn't back from work yet, but he was due home shortly. The three of us sat down and chatted about my operation, and the reconstruction process. Judy praised my great team of doctors, and showed my mom their work on her.

My mom found it difficult to believe that they weren't her own breasts. She couldn't believe how real everything looked, right down to the nipple with the tattooed pigment.

"Well, this certainly makes me feel a lot better," my mom said as she thanked Judy for showing her.

"I'm really worried about my son-in-law," she said. "I know this isn't easy for him either. Perhaps when he sees your outcome, he'll feel as good as I do," she said.

Just then, Randy drove up. He walked in the door and put his brief case down on the floor.

"Sorry, I'm late. The traffic was pretty bad on the freeway," he said.

I introduced Randy to Judy and he thanked her for her willingness to help me throughout the various stages of reconstruction.

"I do this for a lot of people, including husbands and boyfriends of women who are going through this," she said. "I think it's so important for them to see the final results. Pictures don't do justice," she said.

I could tell that Randy was a bit uncomfortable when Judy showed him her breasts, especially in front of his mother-in-law and me. Since this was being done from a medical standpoint, I didn't mind Randy seeing her breasts. Randy agreed with my mother that Judy's breasts looked incredibly real. To this day, I'm extremely grateful to Judy for the complete turn-around Randy made before our eyes.

The next day I was feeling rather courageous and decided to look at my chest in a mirror. Although I was afraid of what I would see, I knew I had to come to terms with it.

I stood in front of the dresser mirror and began unbuttoning my blouse. I slowly slipped the blouse down off my shoulders. I removed the tape that held the gauze in place and gradually unveiled myself. I couldn't help but cry. I looked deformed, disfigured and bruised. Although my chest wasn't completely flat, I was considerably smaller in size (probably a double A or less). I remembered Laurie telling me that the expanders would contain a small amount of saline before they would be surgically implanted.

I looked carefully at the horizontal scars across my breasts where my nipples once were. I was devastated. I could do nothing but cry. I knew I had to mourn the loss of my breasts sooner or later. I just hadn't anticipated falling into such a state of depression, and losing weight like I did as time went on. The depression lasted for several days, up to and including Mother's Day.

I felt too down to go out for Sunday brunch on Mother's Day, but made an effort anyway—mainly for my mother's sake. I hardly ate. I had no appetite.

"Nancy, please eat something," my mom said. "You're thin to begin with. You can't afford to lose any more weight."

"I'm just not hungry," I replied.

Randy began putting things on my plate. Then he held a fork full of hash browns up to my mouth, "Just eat this," he said. I pushed the fork away. I just wanted to go home, crawl in bed, and sleep.

My mom left a few days after Mother's Day. It was sad for me to see her go, as I grew to depend on her help. However, several of our friends and neighbors offered to help us with baby-sitting, cooking, running errands, etc. Fortunately, the depression began to dissipate as I counted the days leading up to May 13, the first expansion.

When I arrived at Dr. Krugman's office for the expansion, Laurie gave me a gown and asked me to lie down on the examination table. She placed a magnet on top of my breast to locate the metal valve inside the expander. When she found the precise location, she took a pen and marked the breast with a dot, and then injected the needle through my skin into the valve. Since I had no sensation in the breast, I didn't feel the needle being inserted.

Next, she pumped the saline through a tube that led to the needle in the expander, until the breast became full. She repeated the process on the opposite breast until it was firm. It was amazing to see my breasts blow up like balloons before my eyes. This was a procedure I came to enjoy. I was gradually gaining back the self-esteem and femininity that I had been stripped of.

My left breast was able to allow 65 cc's of saline before it became firm, while the right radiated breast could only tolerate 50 cc's. This didn't even cause a noticeable difference in the size of each breast, but I became concerned only because the radiated breast couldn't hold the same about of saline. Dr. Krugman said I was doing great and not to worry. If he said I was doing great, then I *was* doing great!

I went for the expansions each week for the first four weeks and then every two weeks thereafter until I reached the desired size. This allowed more time for the skin to stretch and relax between the expansion periods. The right side continued to expand slower than the left side. To compensate, we'd expand only the right breast until it caught up to the amount of saline contained in the left breast.

I went back to work the second week in June and was greeted warmly by my associates. I talked very openly and candidly about my experience with the double mastectomy and what the expansion process entailed. Everyone I spoke to was interested in learning about my experience— especially the reconstructive aspects. I wanted to educate them so they wouldn't feel sorry for me. Moreover, I didn't want them to think that I was terribly disfigured beneath my clothes, like women used to be in year's prior.

To satisfy their curiosity, I'd lean forward and show my cleavage to them. Many of my close friends were totally awestruck, as they knew this was something I never had before and was now extremely proud of. They were so happy to see that I was coming along so nicely, and continued supporting me every step of the way.

In July, I developed a high fever and raspy cough that went on for several days and was getting progressively worse. I went to see my family physician who told me that I had pneumonia! Tears streamed down my face. What next? He put me on antibiotics, and ordered x-rays of my chest, which confirmed I had a mild case of pneumonia. I was thankful that I didn't have to be hospitalized; however, I was laid up for two weeks.

I was extremely disappointed because I was unable to continue with the expansion process until my lungs were clear. Yet another set-back. I certainly didn't expect this to happen, but then again, I never expected to get breast cancer either! By now I was learning that I could handle *anything.*

Toward the end of my recuperation, I decided to see if I could obtain some information from the Internet on the topic of *pregnancy after breast cancer.* I browsed through various breast cancer sites and saw something that caught my eye: *10 Myths About Breast Cancer.* My curiosity got the best of me so I decided to check it out. As I scrolled down the list of myths, I stopped dead in my tracks when I read Myth #7, "*A mastectomy ensures that the cancer is gone forever.*" I couldn't believe my eyes. I re-read it just to make sure I was reading it correctly. There was no mistake. How can this be? The whole idea of women getting mastectomies is to prevent future occurrences. I began to panic as fear set in. Why didn't my doctors tell me this? Is this really true? I couldn't stop thinking about this.

Fortunately, that same day I was scheduled to have a follow-up visit with my family physician who was treating the pneumonia. I told him what I'd read on the Internet. He said that it *is* possible to get cancer again even after a mastectomy, but it's not common. He also said that since I had non-invasive cancer, the chance of a new occurrence was even lower. I felt a sense of relief come over me. He told me not to get caught up in everything I read on the Internet, as that can be dangerous. From then on, I chose not to use the Internet to research any subjects pertaining to breast cancer. It seemed like everything I read lead me to believe that something bad was going to happen, which only made me feel worse.

The doctor told me to have another chest x-ray to ensure my lungs were clear before continuing the expansion process. Fortunately, the x-ray was clear and I could move forward. Laurie continued to track and log the amount of cc's injected into each breast during the expansion sessions, and then she'd take pictures of my breasts at various stages for my file.

I had two goals as far as breast size was concerned, and fortunately Randy agreed with me. 1) I wanted my breasts to be bigger than before, and 2) I wanted them to be proportionate to my small frame. After each expansion, I'd show Randy the results and we'd both agree to "keep going."

My breasts were soon beginning to feel so much pressure from the skin stretching that it was actually causing me pain. Laurie decided to put me on an expansion schedule of every two weeks instead of every week in order to allow more time for the skin to stretch. This seemed to help.

By September I finally reached my goal. Laurie agreed that 450 cc's would be a nice size for me. "You can always change your mind along the way since we'll need to over expand you by 100 cc's per breast."

"Why do I need to be over-expanded by 100 cc's?" I asked.

"So the final results will posture more naturally," she said. "I think you're going to be very pleased with this size. See what your husband thinks and let me know the next time you come in. I'll note it on your chart and we'll go from there," she said.

"Is this a full B or C cup?" I asked.

"Unfortunately, implants aren't ordered by cup size," she said, "they're ordered by the amount of cc's."

"Really? That surprises me."

"Yes. And with the implant manufacturer we use, they only come in increments of 50 cc's."

Before I left, Laurie gave me a packet of information that the implant manufacturer required each patient to read. I was also required to complete and sign several forms, including giving the manufacturer my consent to be monitored every year for five years as part of a study for silicone implants.

That evening when Randy came home from work I showed him my breasts. "Do you think this size is okay?" I asked with my blouse unbuttoned.

"Yes. That's a good size," he said.

"I'm so glad you agree. Now I have to get over expanded by 100 cc's. Laurie said it will make my breasts posture more naturally," I said buttoning up my blouse.

A few weeks later the over-expansion process began. My breasts had gotten so big they were actually annoying me. Every time I moved my arms up, down, or sideways they were there. They were constantly in my way! I even had difficulty sleeping on my sides because my breasts were so big! And, I mean BIG! Well, at least for my frame they were big. By the time I completed the last expansion, none of my clothes fit.

In just a few more weeks, I'd be rid of the uncomfortable expanders, and be made whole again with breasts larger than I initially had! I was counting the days until the operation. October 14, 1998 couldn't come fast enough! I was actually looking forward to having the surgery. I don't know of many who can say that—I must have been the exception! I had waited nearly five months to get to this stage. I was beyond ready.

Dr. Krugman said the operation would be approximately three hours long and would require a general anesthetic. I asked him to put in a request to have Dr. Botzbach as my anesthesiologist again, which he did. He also said I'd need to go on another medical leave for four to six weeks. I made arrangements with my employer and informed my boss of the dates that I would be out of the office. He was very understanding and supportive of what I needed to do.

It was exciting to think that two-thirds of my breast reconstruction soon would be completed. The final stage would encompass the areola and nipple reconstruction—the finishing touches to reclaim my femininity!

12

———

I welcomed the forthcoming surgical implant procedure, and embraced it as though I were going to have a breast augmentation. This was the climax of the reconstructive process, and an exciting opportunity for me to acquire new and improved breasts.

Although this was going to be my fifth surgery, I wasn't the least bit nervous. I had grown accustomed to having operations on my breasts—it was like going to the dentist every six months to get my teeth cleaned!

I was familiar with the "morning of" routine. I'd wake up at 5:15 a.m., take a shower, put on some loose, comfortable clothing, slip on my loafers, and be out the door—all in a matter of 15 minutes. It's amazing how fast a woman can get ready if she doesn't have to put on panty hose, fix her hair, apply make-up, and accessorize!

The sun was just beginning to rise as Randy and I arrived at the hospital. Having been to the hospital so many times, I had become a familiar face to the nursing staff. "Are you here again?" one of the nurses asked as I checked-in.

"Yes. I can't get enough of this place," I said giggling.

"It sure seems that way. Here's some paperwork for you to complete," she said handing me a clipboard and pen. "When you're finished, I'll give you a hospital gown to slip into, and a plastic bag for your belongings."

I sat down next to Randy and began reading and signing all of the necessary documents and medical releases. When I finished, I handed the clipboard back to the nurse.

"Thank you, Nancy," she said handing me a hospital gown and large plastic bag for my clothes. "You can change in there," she said pointing to the restroom.

Once in the gown, I was asked to sit on a gurney so the nurse could take my blood pressure and temperature. I asked her if she knew whether or not Dr. Botzbach was going to be the anesthesiologist.

"Let me check for you." She glanced at some paperwork and replied, "As a matter of fact, she is."

"All right! She's been the anesthesiologist for almost all of my operations. I adore her!" I exclaimed.

Just then, Dr. Krugman entered the room carrying what appeared to be a toolbox. "Don't doctor's carry medical bags anymore?" I asked facetiously. He snickered, opened up the box, and to my surprise, pulled out a level. I was right—it was a toolbox!

"I feel like Tim Allen on the TV show *Home Improvements* every time I do this," he said. Everyone in the room started laughing.

"Is this a joke? Are you really going to use those kinds of tools for this procedure?" I asked.

"Yes, but only prior to going into surgery. I need to be very precise." He asked me to sit upright on the side of the gurney facing a large mirror that was hanging on the wall before me. Randy looked on as Dr. Krugman measured and marked each breast with a pen to ensure both breasts would be level and spaced evenly. I told him exactly how I would like my new breasts to look, and brought in pictures I had cut out of a magazine depicting my expectations.

Just then, Dr. Botzbach entered the room. "I guess I lucked-out again!" I exclaimed. "I'm so glad to have you as the anesthesiologist."

"I wish all of the patients had your enthusiasm," she said humbly.

"So, today you're getting your implants. Is that right?"

"Yes, and I can't wait. I'm so exited to have this operation." "Well then, let's get started."

I laid down on the gurney as she began administering drugs through the I.V. Randy stood beside me, and before I knew it, I was unconscious.

When I awoke I recalled still having had a certain sense of excitement and then remembered why. When I recovered from the anesthesia and was fully alert, I asked one of the nurses if she happened to be in surgery with me.

"Yes, I was," she replied.

"How do I look?" I blurted out referring to my newly found figure.

"You're going to look great in a bathing suit," she said. "They're beautiful."

"Really?"

"Yes, and with your slender figure, you're going to look fabulous!"

What a wonderful compliment, I thought. When I glanced down at my chest, I was surprised to see it tightly wrapped with an ace bandage. I could hardly refrain from unraveling the bandages myself. I was so excited to see what my breasts looked like. The most disappointing part was having drains again—one on each side. I really hated those things!

"You have a post-operative appointment with Dr. Krugman tomorrow at 4 p.m. You can see what your breasts look like then," she said.

"Really? I didn't expect to see them so soon."

"Yes, and be sure not to lift anything for six weeks."

"Okay." I knew that would be a difficult thing to do because I had just grown accustom to lifting and carrying David again during the expansion period.

I got dressed and one of the nurses wheeled me out in a wheelchair. Randy greeted us and helped me get into the car. He cared for me the remainder of the day and night. Randy actually had more responsibility since my mom wasn't there to help out this time. I was impressed with his care-giving abilities—he was excellent! He would make sure I was comfortable, ate something nutritious, and took my pain medication on time. He'd even massage my feet! I couldn't have asked for better care.

My new implants felt so comfortable. Judy had been right! There was no comparison as to how wonderful they felt. Whatever Judy told me to expect, I did—and she was right every step of the way. I don't think Dr. Baick realized what a huge favor he had done for me by introducing me to Judy. Doctors can explain things from a clinical standpoint, but it's not the same as talking to someone who had actually experienced all of the reconstructive stages.

The next day I was ecstatic. I couldn't wait to see my new breasts. My expectations were high to begin with and quickly elevated after hearing the nurse's favorable compliments. I expected to be extremely pleased.

Randy drove me to Dr. Krugman's office. We sat and waited until I was called in. The nurse lead us to an examination room where the "unveiling" was about to take place. The suspense was overwhelming.

I stood while the nurse gradually walked around my body in circles, unwrapping the ace bandage layer by layer. Viola! The bandage was off. I had been staring at Randy's face with excitement the entire time waiting to see his favorable reaction. His face was expressionless. He didn't utter a word. I looked down at my chest. My expectations were shattered. My breasts were swollen and bruised. This isn't what I was supposed to look like! The nurse held a mirror before me as I began to scrutinize further.

"My breasts look smaller than before," I said.

"Perhaps you became accustom to see yourself with larger breasts when the expanders were in. You look great for only one day after surgery," the nurse said.

"I do?" I asked.

"Oh yes. The bruising and swelling is normal. And don't forget you've had this ace bandage wrapped tightly around you since yesterday."

"That's true."

"And look at your cleavage—it's really nice." She did have a point, it was beautiful.

I don't know where on earth my head was. For some reason, I thought the instant the bandages were removed, I'd be walking away looking like a *Playboy* centerfold. I wasn't being realistic. The nurse was right. This was only one day after a three-hour operation. What was I thinking?

When Dr. Krugman came in the examination room, he said that I looked really good for one day post-op. "It's going to take a while before the implants fill out," he said. "In the meantime you need to remain wrapped up in the ace bandage for a total of two weeks. This will prevent the implants from shifting."

It was a nuisance having to be wrapped in an ace bandage 24-hours a-day, but just like everything else, I managed to get through it. Every morning and every night for two weeks, Randy faithfully unwrapped my ace bandage so I could apply ointment on the incisions. Then, he'd tightly wrap me up again. I was beginning to feel like a mummy.

I continued to empty the drains I had on each side—measuring and recording the amount of cc's until it was time for them to be removed.

Every day I was getting better and better and my spirits started to lift. The swelling was going down and the bruises gradually began to fade away. In addition, my breasts were starting to fill out and take on a nice shape, just as Dr. Krugman had said. I felt "at one" with my new breasts; they felt as natural as my real breasts had.

Two weeks later I had my three-month follow-up visit with Dr. Baick. He reviewed my blood test results with me and said everything was normal. When Dr. Baick examined my breasts, he discovered a cyst-like nodule that he believed to be scar tissue along the outer side of the right radiated breast. He suggested that we keep an eye on it and wait six more weeks to see if it would get smaller and gradually go away. That sounded reasonable to me so I didn't become overly concerned.

Right after my appointment with Dr. Baick, I went across the street for my appointment with Dr. Krugman. I showed him the nodule that Dr. Baick had found and he said that he'd keep on eye on it as well. The highlight of the appointment was hearing Dr. Krugman say that I no longer needed to wear the ace bandage, and could finally take a shower. The little milestones meant so much.

While still on a medical leave, I decided to make another appointment with the medical oncologist, Dr. Mahmood. I wanted to get his opinion on whether or not it was safe for me to have another baby now that I'd had a double mastectomy.

As with all of my doctor visits, I came prepared with a list of questions. We had an in-depth and lengthy conversation. It was quite encouraging for me to hear that he thought it was safe for me to have another baby. However, he did suggest that Randy and I wait one year from the time of my double mastectomy to give my body a chance to rest.

In early November, my uncle Sam flew out from Illinois to visit us. He wanted to make sure I was doing well, and spend some time with David, too. Hearing David call him "Grandpa Sam" was music to my ears. David gravitated to my uncle just like he would have to my dad. Imagine my joy.

Uncle Sam and I had some private time to discuss the progress I was making. He was very proud of how well I had handled everything.

"I couldn't have done it without you," I said giving him a big hug. "Oh, stop."

Uncle Sam never liked to take credit for anything. He always gave from the heart and truly enjoyed helping others. He found pleasure in that. I'm proud to tell everyone that I could have never made it this far if it wasn't for the three F's: Faith, Family, and Friends.

By mid-November I was feeling stronger, so Dr. Krugman released me to go back to work. Work was actually good for me. I still enjoyed working three days a week, as it gave me the mental stimulation I needed, as well as the social interaction. My close friends from work were very anxious to see the new me.

One by one, I'd take them into the ladies room and show them my breasts (with my bra on of course—I didn't want them to see me without nipples!) Everyone I showed found them to look unbelievably real. They were all very pleased for me.

Dr. Krugman continued to watch the nodule on my right breast, which hadn't seem to change much, yet it was still there. The doctors suggested that I have an ultrasound to determine exactly what the nodule was. All along, I continued to think it was scar tissue like Dr. Baick speculated. However, since it didn't go away or get smaller I was now beginning to think it may be something else. But, what? It occurred to me that it could be a cancerous lump, but I didn't dwell on that thought. How could one possibly develop breast cancer without breast tissue?

On Monday, December 7, 1998 I went to have an ultrasound on the nodule. After the technician performed the procedure, she asked the radiologist to come in and take a closer look. This isn't a good sign, I thought. I was shocked to see the same radiologist I had had a year ago. His words still remain etched in my brain, "Well, it's definitely not a cyst or clogged milk duct. I suggest you have a biopsy taken." His statement led me to believe that the lump was cancerous. My heart began to race, What is he going to say this time?

"What is it? What do you see?" I asked in a state of panic.

"Well, it's definitely not a tumor. We need to do a biopsy," he said. His words sounded all too familiar.

I threw myself on the examination table, and began sobbing. "I can't go through this again. I just had a double mastectomy to prevent this very thing from happening! Now you're telling me I need a biopsy?! How can this be?! I want to see Dr. Baick right now," I demanded. Then I started to think about the myth I read on the Internet. Maybe mastectomies aren't a cancer cure-all. I had a pretty good history of falling into small categories of rare occurrences and percentages; could this be yet another?

"I'm going to discuss the finding with Dr. Baick," he said. "Please keep your gown on until the technician returns." Alone with my thoughts, I laid on the examination table covering my face with my hands. Hearing the word "biopsy" caused me to panic. I didn't have the wherewithal to go through *another* cancer ordeal. The longer I waited in the examination room, the more convinced I became that I had cancer again. This time I may not get off as easy, I thought. I may need to undergo chemotherapy. Oh my God!

Soon, the technician came back and took me to an examination room where I waited for Dr. Baick. Margo, his nurse, came in to see me. I started crying and she gave me a big hug.

"You'll feel better when you talk to Dr. Baick," she said.

"I hope you're right," I said wiping away my tears. "I can't take much more."

When Dr. Baick entered the room he immediately looked at the nodule.

"I don't think this is anything to worry about—it could just be subcutaneous fat. However, I'm going to do a needle biopsy right now."

The nurse handed him a large needle. He lifted the nodule up and away from the implant so as not to puncture it. He injected a rather large needle into the nodule extracting fluid. Fortunately, it was painless as I had no sensation in that particular area of the breast.

"We'll have the biopsy results for you on Thursday. However, I still want to schedule you for surgery on Friday and have it removed," he said. "The good thing is that we'll know what it is going into surgery. Either way, we need to take it out."

I was beside myself. What next? I drove home and waited for Randy to arrive from work. When he did, I explained what happened, and how I was going to have to undergo another surgery.

"Nancy, you're going to be fine. If it will make you feel better, call Dr. Debbie and get her opinion," he said.

"Great idea."

Fortunately she was home when I called. Since she was my doctor friend, I'd shared all of my progress with her. I explained the new turn of events.

"What do you think it could be Deb?" I asked.

"I think you're doctor's probably right. Don't worry. It can't be anything else because your breast tissue has already been removed."

"Can you think of anything strange that it could possibly be? I seem to fall into rare and unusual categories," I said, trying to make light of the situation.

"Well the chances are slim—like five percent, but it could be a reactive lymph node."

"What does that mean?" I asked.

"Well, your body could have created a reaction in one of the lymph nodes just from the surgeries, or as a reaction to the implant. You're probably just more concerned because it's on the radiated side, right?"

"Yes," I said.

"Don't worry, it's nothing to get upset over."

The next few days at work were difficult. As much as I wanted to believe that things were going to be alright, I had this gnawing feeling in my stomach that perhaps it might not be.

While having lunch with Marcia, Laura, and Maria, I decided to tell them about the most recent medical encounter. I began to sob as I shared my never-ending frustrations. Marcia grabbed my hand and held it tightly, reassuring me that I was going to be okay. I could see the sorrow in each of their eyes.

On Wednesday, someone from Dr. Baick's office called to tell me that the biopsy was negative—Praise God! The pathology report indicated it was a reactive lymph node with fatty tissue—nothing serious, but still another rare finding! Having this information prior to the surgery made me feel much more at ease.

Since Randy was away on business, my brother offered to take me to the hospital at 6 a.m. on Friday. Fortunately, our baby sitter was able to come to the house as early as 5:45 a.m. This wasn't going to be a major operation, but nonetheless, it was yet another surgery that I didn't eagerly anticipate.

I was in surgery for less than 45 minutes, and since it was a local anesthetic I recovered rather quickly. I was relieved to know that I had only one more surgery until the reconstructive process was complete—unless of course, I ran into another hiccup along the way!

13

On January 20, 1999—just two days before my 38th birthday, I had the last of a total of seven operations on my breasts. The surgery was to create the nipples and the areolas by taking skin from my lower abdomen.

This reconstructive procedure is ingenious. Try to envision a woman's areola. Imagine cutting a semi-circle horizontally across the lower half, lifting the skin up and over, then bunching it together to form a nipple. To replace the semi-circle of skin used to form the nipple, skin is taken from the lower abdomen in the shape of an ellipse. I wasn't upset about having an incision in my lower abdomen, because Dr. Krugman was going to use the incision from the Cesarean section I had when I delivered David.

Randy and I were elated that this two-year ordeal would soon be over. We were ready to move on to the next chapter in our lives.

When we arrived at the hospital I went through the customary procedures of completing all of the forms and signing the releases. Before I knew it, I was once again sitting on the side of a gurney in a hospital gown waiting for Dr. Krugman to arrive. He told me that prior to going into surgery I'd have the opportunity to choose a rubber template depicting the size of the areola and the nipple I preferred. How nice to be able to have choices in such things!

Upon Dr. Krugman's arrival, he began marking the sites of the areola and nipple on each breast. I chose an areola template large enough to cover the incision from where my areolas and nipples previously were. Randy looked on and was included in the decision. Dr. Krugman reiterated that he had to be extra careful on the radiated breast.

The next person to enter the room was the anesthesiologist, Dr. Botzbach. Once again I was overjoyed to know that she would be with me during surgery. Since she was the anesthesiologist for almost all of my operations, we became quite friendly.

"This is the last time you're going to see me," I said jokingly.

"I hope so," she said. "Well, I didn't mean that how it sounded. I just meant that I didn't want you to have to go through any more procedures," she said chuckling.

"I understood what you meant. Just don't be surprised if I request to have you as the anesthesiologist when I deliver our next baby."

"I would be honored," she said.

By this time the nurses had me hooked up to an I.V. so Dr. Botzbach could begin administering the anesthetics. Randy stood at my side as I was wheeled into the operating room.

Since I had a local anesthetic, as opposed to a general, it was much easier to recover. When I awoke from the surgery, there were two large, clear plastic domes covering each breast. Adhered to each dome were several yellow and orange happy face stickers. I started laughing. I think the nurses were happy for me too, as they knew it was my last operation.

My next appointment with Dr. Krugman was one week away. The nurse said the domes were designed to protect the nipples from collapsing in the event that I was jarred. I was required to wear the domes for four weeks. It sounded rather long, but it was a better trade-off than having to contend with tubes and drains!

When I finished dressing, one of the nurses wheeled me outside as we waited for Randy to drive up. I was amazed that I able to get out of the wheel chair and into the car with minimal assistance.

I spent the majority of the next few days sleeping. For some reason, I expected the pain in my breasts to be greater than the pain in my lower abdomen, but it was just the opposite. To my surprise my lower abdomen hurt more—almost as much as having a Cesarean. It was awful.

I was determined not to spend my birthday in bed. Randy offered to take me out to dinner if I felt up to it. In preparation for that, I took two naps; one in the morning and one in the afternoon. I wanted to store up enough energy to get out of the house—even if it was just for an hour.

Early in the afternoon, Shari, my cousin's wife, called. "Are you feeling up to having some visitors this evening?" she asked.

"Absolutely. What time did you have in mind?"

"Oh, about 5 p.m. John and Sue would like to drive up from San Diego to see you too," she said. John and Sue are my godparents from Wisconsin, who spend their winters in San Diego.

"That would be great, because Randy and I have dinner reservations at 7 p.m."

"We won't stay long. We have plans to go to the theater tonight."

Shortly after 5 p.m., Shari and my godparents arrived with a birthday cake in their hands. "Happy Birthday!" they shouted in unison.

"Thank you. That's nice of you to remember."

"You look so good," said Shari.

"You really do," said Sue.

"We're glad that this is all behind you, and admire your positive attitude," said John.

"Gee thanks. I don't know how to react to all of these wonderful compliments," I said blushing.

Just then the doorbell rang—it was Tod. "Happy Birthday!" he said giving me a kiss on the cheek. I enjoyed having the house filled with family and relatives, especially on my birthday.

A few minutes later, Randy arrived carrying a cake, "Happy Birthday Honey!" he said handing me the cake, and giving me a kiss.

"Wow, now I have two birthday cakes!" I exclaimed.

"One for each side," he said snickering.

"And double the wishes!"

Everyone sang Happy Birthday, including David, while I made a wish and blew out the candles. Randy served the cake, and before we knew it, it was time for the relatives to leave.

Tod had previously offered to tend to David so Randy and I could go out for dinner. Randy took me to a restaurant in Laguna Beach, about 30 minutes away. We had a nice romantic dinner at a charming little restaurant. During dinner he presented me with a small velvet box. "This is for your birthday," he said leaning over to kiss me, "and to celebrate the end of all your surgeries. You made it!"

I had a feeling it might be the diamond cocktail ring that I had my eye on for several months, but I didn't know for sure. I slowly opened the box and looked inside.

"You got it for me!" I exclaimed. "I love it! Thank you, thank you, thank you!"

"I knew you how much you liked it when you saw it at the store. I wanted you to have it."

"Randy," I said, "I couldn't have made it without you."

"Sure you could have. You have what it takes. That's why I married you." He slipped the ring on my finger. It fit perfectly!

"This is one of my most memorable birthdays," I said smiling ear to ear. "And I have you to thank."

Toward the end of the month, Dr. Krugman took off the bandages so I could finally see what the areolas and nipples looked like. I watched closely as he removed the bandages with tweezers. I literally cried tears of joy upon seeing them.

"They're beautiful!" I exclaimed, wiping away my tears. "Thank you Dr. Krugman."

"If you think they look good now, just wait another few weeks and you'll really be pleased," the nurse said.

"You'll need to wear the domes for three more weeks and be very careful. Any major trauma to the breast could cause the nipples to collapse," Dr. Krugman said.

"How soon do you think they'll be able to begin the tattooing process?" I asked.

"Probably some time in early March," he said. "I'll set you up with Christine, who we use to tattoo the pigment for areolas and nipples."

During the following weeks I was very protective of my chest—especially around David, a typical toddler, who loves running around and charging into people. Each week I saw a major difference in my nipples. They were starting to heal and take on a realistic appearance. I was thrilled! I was beginning to feel whole again.

I remember Judy saying, "Just wait until you get your tattoos. That's the finishing touch." I longed for the day I would be totally complete—and to think it was just around the corner.

I went back to work in mid-February, and was quite anxious to show off my breasts now that the reconstruction was complete. Showing my new breasts to other women was like showing them a new dress I bought. It was that simple!

By early March, Dr. Krugman said it was time to get the areolas and nipples tattooed. He suggested I set up an appointment with Christine, an intradermal cosmetic technician who specialized in pigment color technology.

Dr. Krugman had previously explained to Christine that my right breast had been radiated and the skin was very thin. To avoid any risk of damaging the implant during the tattooing process, he instructed her to be extremely careful.

Christine had never applied color to a patient with a radiated breast before, but that didn't bother me. It was rare for a woman to have reconstruction after radiation, so I expected her not to have any experience in that area. She showed me the electric tool she would be using, which looked and sounded similar to a dentist's electric drill.

"Since the right side has been radiated, I won't be able to punch-in the pigment like I'm going to do on the left side. I don't want to risk puncturing your implant. Instead, I'm going to draw on the pigment," she said. "It's not as permanent and may fade quicker."

The process took approximately one hour. During that time she told me that she was a breast cancer survivor as well. "That's how I got into this business," she said. "I had a simple mastectomy and just made my five-year anniversary on November 22nd."

"You're kidding. That's my anniversary date too; well, it was for my first bout with breast cancer," I said. "Now that I've had a double mastectomy, the anniversary date changed to April 24th."

I learned that anniversary dates for cancer survivors are just as important as birthdays—you can't forget them, and you always celebrate them.

The procedure didn't hurt much. I felt a bit of pain in the areas where I still had some sensitivity. After she finished, I looked down at myself in complete awe. This was the icing on the cake.

"They look so good!" I exclaimed.

"Don't they? You'll have to come back in a few weeks so I can treat the area again. It provides for better coverage," she said. "You won't be able to take a shower for five days and you'll need to apply this ointment three times a day for five days," she said handing me some sample packets.

"Oh no, not again. I thought the days of not being allowed to take showers were over," I said.

"Almost over," she replied.

When Randy came home from work that evening, I told him how happy I was and showed him my breasts.

"Nancy, if I didn't know better, I would have thought they were real," he said.

"I know. I'm just so pleased."

Having these breasts made me feel like a new woman. I couldn't wait to go out and buy some new tops—tight ones, with plunging necklines. I felt wonderful. More confident. More feminine. I felt like I had the world at my fingertips. And I did—with an entirely new appreciation for life, and all of God's beautiful gifts.

Those who know me have witnessed my ability to develop courage in times of desperation. They were amazed at my refusal to wallow in self-pity, taking heed as I embraced blow after blow open-handedly.

How did I manage to do this? I didn't run or hide from the fear—I faced it. Facing fear is how I grew. And, it became easier and easier the more I put it to use. This tactic, combined with my faith in God, became my saving grace and proved to be invaluable.

I too, saw myself becoming a stronger person with each hardship I endured—beginning with the death of my father. His death laid the foundation on which I built my stamina. I knew that if I could learn to accept the loss of my father, I could learn to accept just about anything.

Today my friends refer to me as a "warrior" and a "hero". I think it's a bit overstated, but nonetheless, I smile and thank them for their compliment.

I learned a lot about myself through this journey of surgeries and life-altering decisions. I discovered that I have a strong network of family and friends who I can rely on. I have seen my priorities change, and now I have a better understanding of what's really important to me. Although I'm cancer-free, the experience has touched my life and become a part of who I am.

It was a journey that I'll never forget—a journey I feel privileged to have taken.

Epilogue

After returning home from the appointment with Christine, I read an article in the newspaper stating that a reorganization was going to take place at the company I was employed by. It stated that 1,400 positions worldwide were going to be eliminated. Good grief! Perhaps my job is in jeopardy I thought—especially since I'm only working part-time.

I had heard rumors of this possibility but didn't think twice about it. I knew the corporation had a history of being extremely sound and profitable. According to the article, the lay-offs were to occur on Monday. Since Monday was not my scheduled workday, I was curious as to how this would be handled, if indeed I were to be let go.

The following day was Friday, my scheduled day off. To my dismay, I received a telephone call at home from the secretary in our department saying there was a mandatory meeting at noon on Monday. I was advised to attend. At this point I knew my job was history.

"Maybe that's a good thing," Randy said. "You won't have any work-related stress anymore, and you can spend even more time with David. You can always find another part-time job if you want to. Besides, you still don't know for sure. You're just speculating."

By this time, I had been with the company for more than 12 years. I grew up there. I couldn't imagine working anywhere else. I was just at the point where I was getting normalcy restored to my life, and now this.

I recalled how, during my struggles with breast cancer, my dear friend Kathryn taught me to believe that *everything is as it should be*. I soon came to realize that I had developed strong mental capabilities from my breast cancer experiences, which enabled me to learn to cope with *any* situation—even a potential lay-off. And, the beauty of it is, I can share it with others.

On Monday I reported to work an hour ahead of schedule. The atmosphere was drastically different from the fast-paced environment I grown to know over the years. It was strangely eerie and depressing. And for a good reason. Many of the employees were nervous and fearful of losing their jobs, myself included; but I was prepared. Shortly after noon, my boss called me into his office. It was obvious. I was going to lose my job.

"I hate to do this to you Nancy," he said, "but your position has been eliminated."

"I figured it would be, being part-time and all."

"I want you to realize that this has nothing to do with your performance. Your job has just been eliminated due to the reorganization. We certainly appreciate all of your years of loyal service," he said.

"Well, I appreciate you giving me the opportunity to work in a part time capacity this past year and a half. It was really great," I said.

"This is a very difficult thing for me to do. You're certainly making it a lot easier by being so composed."

"I've survived cancer two times. I certainly can survive a lay-off. This by far is nothing in comparison," I said.

"Take this time and think about what you really want to do. Now is your chance to fulfill your dreams." Perhaps he's right, I thought.

He went over the severance package with me. As part of the package, each associate was given an opportunity to attend a two-day career transition seminar conducted by a professional out-placement services provider. Rick thought it would be helpful and encouraged me to go.

I turned over my corporate ID badge to Rick, and sadly started packing my belongings. Throughout the day, one by one I saw many of my colleagues walking out the door with their boxes of belongings. Some left in tears. It was a dark day. I kept reminding myself that I was *alive,* and healthy, and being laid-off was nothing in comparison to what I had endured in my battle with cancer.

I decided to attend the two-day workshop, which proved to be very beneficial. The first day of class, one of the trainers had us participate in an exercise. She asked each of us to close our eyes and turn the clock ahead ten years. "Envision where you are, and what you're doing," she said. For approximately five minutes, the room was completely silent. Each of us sitting quietly with our eyes closed.

When I closed my eyes I saw myself at a popular bookstore where a book-signing event was taking place. Crowds of people gathered, forming a large line around a small banquet-size table. People were waiting in line to meet the author and get an autographed copy of her book. The author sitting behind the table was ME!

I don't have to wait ten years for that to happen, I thought. I can make it happen now. I've always dreamed of someday writing a book, and now I have a great story to tell. I'm going to do it!

"Facing Fear: A Young Woman's Personal Account of Surviving Breast Cancer," was soon underway. It was an opportunity for me to reach out and tell my story. I wanted young women and their families to be educated, inspired, and learn that life's challenges can only be met with an abundance of perseverance.

If I hadn't been laid-off, I would have never made a shift in my career to become an author. And, if I hadn't experienced a bout with breast cancer, I could have never written this book nor been able to share my experience with you.

You see, *everything is as it should be.*

Life. It does find ways to complete a circle, allowing us to move forward again. On August 5, 1999, what would have been my father's

74th birthday, Randy and I received another blessing from God. We're expecting our second baby in April 2000.

Our prayers have once again been answered and our lives continue to become enriched in ways we can only imagine…

Perspectives

Personal thoughts from those closest to me....

From a Husband's Point of View
by Randy Madey

Finding out your wife has cancer is not something you anticipate, plan on or talk about in home economics class. You quickly have to embrace this ugly feeling of "this isn't really happening, right?" You ask "why" several times, and then wonder what in the world could have triggered such a thing? When? How on earth did this manifest itself inside the woman I love?

I remember getting that first call while I was away on business, telling me my wife had a strong possibility of having breast cancer and needed surgery. I was stunned. I thought the biopsy was just a precaution the doctor used to rule out cancer. Fortunately, I was able to return from my business trip in time for her surgery.

While at the hospital, I was confident everything would be okay, but there was still doubt in the back of my mind. The worst part of the whole process was not the operation, but waiting four days for the lab results.

You really have to give up control and turn worry into positive thoughts. So when waiting for lab results, there is nothing you can do but distract yourself from the issues at hand. Nancy and I found that movies were a good diversion. And just hearing our son's laughter at play made all the painful thoughts go away temporarily.

When the pathology report confirmed the lump to be cancerous, it was devastating! No one likes bad news. So now what?

One could spend months consulting specialists, getting second and third opinions, trying to determine the best course of action. Advice from friends and family were helpful, but it came down to what was comfortable for us, and more importantly, Nancy. She had the final decision as to the type of treatment she was willing to endure. Based on the doctor's recommendation, we decided to choose radiation therapy as a preventative measure against a reoccurrence.

The most painful experience came sixteen months later. Nancy called me at work to tell me the results of her first annual mammogram after surviving cancer. She said the mammogram on her opposite breast looked suspicious, possibly cancer. I certainly did not know what to think, and feared the worst. I asked to talk with the doctor. I needed details; a glimmer of hope that this was something minor. The thought of being without Nancy flashed through my mind. What would I do? What about our son? Dr. Baick gave me more information and reassured me early detection was a positive thing.

Going to the doctor's office to get the results of the biopsy was tough. Waiting was even harder this time. We wanted the biopsy results to be clean. I certainly did not expect to walk out thinking a double mastectomy was going to be an option. But this was a way to remove the possibility of future occurrences. I reassured Nancy that I would be there for her during the process and love her just the same.

A mastectomy could have an impact on a marriage. There is your wife's feelings of loss, and dealing with those feelings *together* is critical in the acceptance of the entire process. Being supportive and letting Nancy know that the new breast "tissue" didn't make her less desirable was probably the most important reassurance I could give her. I felt she needed to have an unconditional acceptance of her new body. I believed that if Nancy knew I accepted her, it would help her healing process. And it did. Although she had her moments of sadness, she was able to overcome them in a way I never dreamed of. I'm extremely proud of her, and proud to have her as my wife.

Having our faith and believing a higher power was looking out for us helped ease the pain.

I don't think I'll ever forget this experience and how we both gained strength from it.

From a Mother's Point of View
by Alice Mikaelian

Can you imagine having just lost your husband to cancer and then being told that your youngest daughter has breast cancer? The thought of losing her was absolutely devastating.

I had flown to California to be with my daughter, her husband, and my dear grandchild for Thanksgiving, only to be told she has breast cancer, and just had had a lumpectomy the day before.

How I wish my husband were here to comfort me—I felt so alone. Of course, this would have torn him apart since she was the apple of his eye.

Nancy was very optimistic. She said the cancer was caught early and everything was going to be fine. She was so brave. I was so proud of her. She said she would get through this, and I wanted to believe her.

My emotions let lose every night when I was alone. I didn't want her to know my feelings. As a mother, I traveled back and forth from Wisconsin to California just to be near her at this critical time.

I was there for her radiation treatments and then throughout most of the surgeries that followed. You see, just shortly after a year, cancer developed in her opposite breast, resulting in a double mastectomy. Breast cancer at the age of 35. Then, at the young age of 37, with a child two years old, she had to undergo more surgeries.

I thank the Lord for the final outcome. She is a beautiful young woman with a good outlook on life. And she is looking forward to having another baby. She's put the breast cancer behind her and is going on with her life.

Our prayers have been answered.

From a Brother's Point of View
by Tod C. Mikaelian

I clearly remember the day my mom and dad came home from the hospital with my new baby sister. I ran all the way home from school just to see her. It was a day of great joy.

Thirty-five years later, I find out that she has breast cancer. It's a day I don't like to recall.

As her brother, I'm not sure how much support I gave her; however, I tried the best I could. As difficult as it was for me, I couldn't even begin to imagine what it was like for Nancy—especially after just becoming a mother.

Hearing that she had a new occurrence a little over a year later was even more shocking and devastating than the first time! I knew how hard Nancy fought. She was so *positive* and brave—only to get slapped down again. I remember how my stomach churned the morning she called to tell me.

Although she still focused on the hopeful aspects, there were days when reality would hit her. I recall one evening on the phone when she was feeling really down. I found myself feeling her pain, yet not knowing what to say or how to comfort her. I was at a loss for words and it bothered me all night.

The next day, I called David Dukes, the president and COO of the company where both Nancy and I worked, and arranged to speak with him. David is very positive and a very motivating man whom both Nancy and I admire. I told him about Nancy's new finding, and asked if he could give her a call and talk to her. I felt he could make a difference. David was more than willing.

A few hours later he walked back to my office to tell me that he spoke to my sister, and they had a good talk. He said she'd be fine. I was very grateful that he did that for me.

It seemed from that point on, Nancy took her illness and was determined not to let it take her down. I'm truly amazed at how she has fought this.

I love my sister dearly. At times when I didn't have the words to say, I knew that a hug from her brother was all that she needed.

From a Sister's Point of View
by Kathy Merrick

My little sister has breast cancer—no, it can't be true. How could this happen to her? If she dies, I'll want to die, too. Tears stream down my face. She's just got to be okay. She undergoes a lumpectomy and is told she needs radiation treatments that will last several weeks. I pray she'll be all right.

In March, the following year, I visit Nancy in California and she asks me to accompany her to her mammogram appointment. I'm actually with her when the doctor tells her he sees something suspicious on her x-rays.

We follow the doctor to another room and he shows us the x-ray. The calcifications in question look like specks of dust even when magnified. This can't be cancer, I think. I'm leaving my sister tomorrow afternoon to return home to Colorado. I feel I need to be with her, although I know there is nothing I can do. It's in God's hands.

The day Nancy has her appointment with her doctor to find out her biopsy results, I call her physician's office knowing she is there with Randy. They refuse to tell me anything. When I finally do reach my sister, she tells me it's cancer. She will opt to have a double mastectomy in April. I cry a lot at first and later just try to erase this nightmare from my mind.

As her day of surgery arrives, I'm nervous, distraught, and very stressed out. She's got to be okay—poor kid. She doesn't deserve this. The day drags on endlessly.

In the many months that follow, she goes through several reconstructive surgeries. She tells me she's happy with the results, but I have this haunting fear that she will die sooner than I do.

The fear causes me pain because she's my little sister, the sister I love so much.

From a Best Friend's Point of View
By Mary Laros

I first found out that my best friend Nancy had cancer through a phone call I received from our mutual friend, Sandi. I remember listening to Sandi tell me that Nancy was diagnosed with breast cancer. My mind raced with incredible thoughts. I was speechless! After all, the mere mention of the word "cancer" is frightening.

I had my first experience with cancer five years ago when my father was diagnosed with adencarcinoma. I watched helplessly as he suffered a long and painful death. It's an experience that my mind and heart will never forget.

Unfortunately, the time came again for me to think about cancer. How could this be? Had the doctors made a mistake? She's only 35 years old!

I took a deep breath, anxiously looking for Nancy's telephone number. I kept telling myself I needed to be strong and supportive for my dear friend. I made the phone call and Nancy explained everything to me. She was so strong and optimistic—it was as if she were supporting me.

A series of phone calls began back and forth to one another. I wished I could have done more. I felt sad and helpless once again. Above all, I wished we lived closer so I could hug her, love her, and assure her it was going to be okay.

Of course, one tends to question his or her own mortality when hearing about such life-threatening situations. I prayed a lot and lit

several candles in church for the dear Lord to hear my prayers and save my friend.

As time went on, things managed to quite down and life continued. However, I constantly thought about Nancy.

Nancy had mentioned that her annual mammogram was coming up. She hoped that there wasn't going to be any surprises this time. Little did we know, she had a suspicious-looking mammogram showing more cancer.

This time when I heard the news I was shaking. I listened quietly and tried to be brave. I couldn't comprehend that my friend of 23 years, who was young and healthy, had cancer for the second time. I looked to friends and family for support. I was concerned about what was going to happen next. Our weekly phone calls began once again. *I* needed to have Nancy keep me informed on her prognosis, however, I didn't want to become a nuisance. I knew that she had repeated the same story to family and friends enough times. Yet, it was very important to me that she know I cared.

When I wasn't home, Nancy would leave me positive messages on my answering machine. I can remember falling back on my bed and rejoicing with tears in my eyes. Thanking God for His blessings.

Last summer, after Nancy's double mastectomy, we were finally able to get together. It was wonderful—we sobbed and rejoiced like sisters and cried. It was a feeling of pure happiness—sharing an intuitive sense of what we were both feeling.

I wish my loving friend a life of health, love and joy. After all, she's a mother, daughter, wife, sister, and *my* best friend!

From Kathryn's Point of View
by Kathryn A. Mitchell

I liked Nancy Mikaelian Madey the first time I met her. Now I love her.

When Nancy first came to me about 12 years ago (we worked for the same company), she impressed me as being a warm, caring soul, with a dazzling personality. I was drawn to her cheerfulness and effervescence. She was stunning, with long, black curly hair, large brown puppy-like eyes, and an enviable figure.

As our friendship grew over the years, I began to notice a metamorphosis taking place in my young friend. It seemed to start with the event of her beloved father's death. Oh, how devastating this was for Nancy. She mourned so deeply that she was truly inconsolable. There was nothing that would bring her through her pain. Nancy grieved on, and on and on, unable or unwilling to let go.

Then, Nancy was dealt another cruel blow. She was diagnosed with breast cancer. When she first told me about it, my initial thoughts were that this girl could never get through the impending tribulations. I did not see her as having the strength and fortitude to face the ordeal she was about to encounter. If Nancy could not get over the passing of her father after several years, how could she deal with the fact of her own mortality?

Never underestimate the powers of the mind and of the spirit.

I didn't know it at the time, but I was about to become witness to the birth of a beautiful butterfly. After the initial shock and panic of the news about her health, Nancy slowly came to grips with the situation and faced it head-on. I watched Nancy grow from a self-pitying girl into a magnanimous woman. The changes were slow and often painful in Nancy's development, but they nonetheless came about surely and truly.

One of the most difficult accomplishments of Nancy's breast cancer experience was maintaining her cheerfulness and optimism. Before her battle ended, she would endure seven surgeries! She developed the courage and strength to face it all with the healthiest of attitudes imaginable. Of course, Nancy had her moments with pain, fear, depression and the elements of the unknown which tormented her. But her overall demeanor remained truly remarkable in that she forced herself to change her attitude. She stopped seeing herself as simply a victim of an evil quirk of fate. Instead, she began to see her experience as a learning process that could bring benefit to herself and others who may face the horrors of finding out they have cancer. She started to recognize opportunities to broaden her own horizons through her journey down the long road to recovery, and acted bravely upon every one of them.

Now that Nancy has told her touching story, *Facing Fear: A Young Woman's Personal Account of Surviving Breast Cancer*, I think she is one of the richest people I know. And I am certainly richer for having Nancy in my life.